THE
ANTI-DIET

How To Eat, Lose, and Live

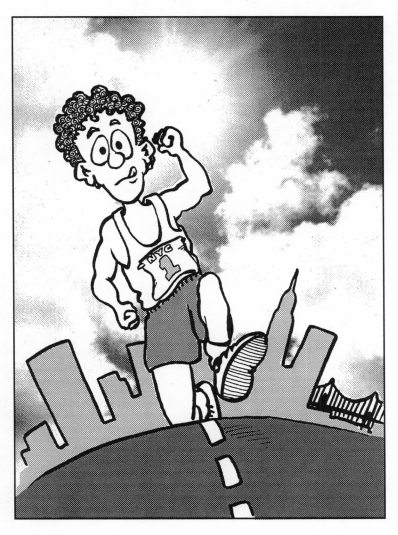

by
Mickey Harpaz, Ph.D.

Aitan Publishing Co.
c/o Benay Enterprises, Inc.
62 East Starrs Plain Road
Danbury, CT 06810

Text © 1996 Mickey Harpaz, Ph.D.
Cover Design © 1996 Terrie Dunkelberger
Book Design and Illustrations © 1996 Paul Gordon

paper ISBN: 0-9650782-0-5

0   9   8   7   6   5   4   3   2   1

Dedication

This book is dedicated to the inner strength of my family;
To my wife Jill and to my children, Aitan and Koren --
the highest motivations I have ever had to create my healthy
lifestyle. I love you.

THE ANTI-DIET:
How to Eat, Lose, and Live

CONTENTS

Acknowledgments

I am immeasurably indebted to my managers and advocates Neil Reshen and Dawn Reshen-Doty of Benay Enterprises, Inc. Their intelligence, experience, insight, and patience are everything an author could ask for.

My special thanks to my editor Patiricia Allen for her careful examination of my text for language accuracy, clarity, and completeness. Her on-going efforts have been extraordinary and her feedback invaluable.

My appreciation and admiration to my illustrator Paul Gordon who graciously and humorously provided fun days which will not be forgotten. Paul, you are a genius at work.

I gratefully acknowledge my debt to Mike McGetrick, William and Judy Riebe whose faith in me provided strong support and allowed this project to be completed.

Last but not least, my profound thanks and love to my parents Pnina and David Harpaz. This book would not have been possible without you.

Author's Note:

This book is not a substitute for conventional medical treatment; it is a supplement to medical treatment. If you have heart problems (i.e. coronary heart disease), have elevated cholesterol, high blood pressure or diabetes, or if you are obese or have any other health problem, you must consult your physician before beginning any type of diet or exercise program or before trying to implement the program in this book.

Every person is different. Heredity and lifestyle can affect the outcome of any nutritional and exercise program. Only after consulting your physician and/or other health care professional can you make decisions affecting your own health.

If you are taking any medication, your physician may wish to decrease or discontinue some or all such medication if your clinical status improves. As your condition improves and you lose weight, your clinical status may change. Your cholesterol, blood glucose level, or blood pressure may change. These changes may help you reduce your medication dosage or eliminate the need for it altogether. However, do not make any changes in your medication without consulting your doctor first.

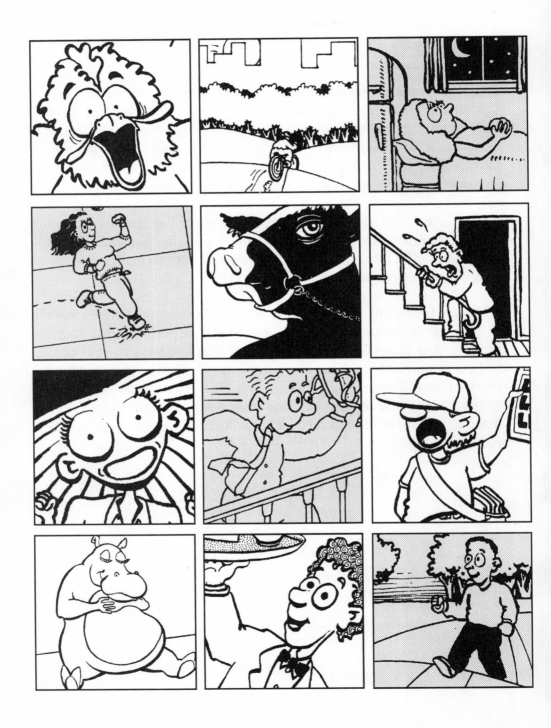

Introduction

Welcome to the Anti-Diet program. As a health consultant with a degree in exercise physiology and nutrition, I look forward to sharing with you the most current information I have to help you stop dieting endlessly, stop wasting your money on diets, and start living a normal and healthy life. All you have to do is to read this book, take notes, and implement the Anti-Diet program one step at a time.

First, however, let me congratulate you for making two very wise decisions: (1) to stop the yo-yo dieting syndrome and (2) to step into a normal and healthy lifestyle. Let us all understand that this book is written for most of us—people like you and me who have become obsessed with diets.

My goal in writing this book is to help increase your understanding of lifestyle changes, lifestyle choices, and how they can affect your health, your conditioning, and your general well-being. This is really much more than just a weight loss book. I am an exercise physiologist and a nutritionist, that is a specialist in helping people change their lifestyles—a specialist in helping people to build up a nourishing diet based on proper eating habits and proper nutrition.

But this book will not only help you improve your health and well-being, it will enable you to enhance your ability to metabalize food, strengthen your immune system, and, at the same time, increase your energy level. In addition it can really help you lose weight *without deprivation or hunger.*

The Anti-Diet program is an invitation to change a life-long habit of dieting into a life-affirming choice for good health by:

- Building and maintaining a vital metabolism
- Increasing daily activity and exercise
- Learning core proper eating habits
- Integrating the latest nutritional facts into a common sense eating lifestyle that increases energy and over all health

With the *Anti-Diet* program you will never *ever* fall into the trap of dieting again!

Aside from helping you lose weight and keep it off, this book is a supplement to prevention treatments for heart disease, obesity, osteoporosis, diabetes, colon cancer, prostate cancer, breast cancer, stroke, hypertension, hypercholesterolemia and many other illnesses. The Anti-Diet program is based upon scientific studies that have been published in many professional journals. My goal is to outline, in simple terms the workings of physiology and nutrition, and to show how the two combine to implement a correct lifestyle: a lifestyle that makes sense, that won't leave you feeling deprived or hungry, and a lifestyle that will provide you with plenty of energy. Eventually, you will stop talking, living, thinking, and breathing diets and weight loss.

At this point I'd like very much to share my own story with you. My romance with food started a long time ago. Digging deeply into my memory, to the time I was four or five years old, a frightening thought takes over: I should have weighed 300 pounds by now. My life was surrounded by one profound, major activity: EATING! Eating, food, meals, family events, holidays and mostly Mom's cooking. God bless her—what a cook!

I can remember the social hierarchy in my house. My mother would be cooking, and my father would be eating—at any given time. Of course, my dad says, "We cooked, we ate, we enjoyed the food." Remarkably enough, on 95% of those occasions, my mom never tasted her own cooking. Bread, cheese, and olives were her most usual intake for the day.

One of the major social rules in my house was "the 7:00 p.m. dinner." Dinnertime was wartime in my house. First, back at home in Israel, you never knew when the next war would be triggered. Sit, eat, and finish fast. If the war arrives on your doorstep, you won't have to fight hungry! Second, no incoming/outgoing phone calls—no communication with the outside world. Third, forget *Archie* and *Soap*—no TV. Enjoy the taste, smell and color of the food. At dinnertime we enjoyed good family conversations, solved personal problems, and spent much less money on psychological counseling.

My dad's love for food and capacity for food consumption astonished me. This person, on his good days, consumed the equivalent of an entire army unit's "mess" in an afternoon. I recall a ceremonial pre-dinner meal on Firday afternoons. Dad used to sit with a pitcher of tea, 2.5 to 4.5 pounds of oranges, and a Hallah bread cut in half and filled with butter and honey. Consuming this snack prepared him for the 7:00 p.m. Friday Jewish dinner, which in itself can put a Thanksgiving dinner to shame.

Mom, on the other hand, never ate a lot. However, her combat history as a fitness instructor in the Palmach, training guys to stand against the British Mandate, was transferred directly to the kitchen and the dining table. First, there was never a problem about inviting a friend over for dinner. Although there were only three of us in the house, Mom, did not eat her own food, still thought we were in the army. So the quantities were big enough to feed our entire block. Second, you could never dare say "no" to a second serving. Her sergeant's glare and the guilt trip she imposed on you were enough to force you to ask for a third serving. Last, there were times when I was bold enough, or perhaps just not smart enough, when a request for a little more came from my mouth. The smile of happiness on Mom's face made it appear as though she had hit her target and captured the enemy. My punishment—a whopping portion that could pass as a meal in itself. But with Mom as cook, I never said "no."

During my school years, I had another tough customer to deal with. Grandma. Sometimes I wondered who took lessons from whom; Mom from Grandma, or vice versa. However, as I grew, I recognized that my Grandma used a different strategy. A visit to her house was a trip to bribery land. I visited my aging Grandma on a regular basis to help her with the daily chores. With years of experience, she knew how to bribe me into staying longer by serving the types of foods that only a grandma would cook for her grandson. Soon my visits became longer and closer to dinnertime at home. The situation literally became too big for me to handle, and the only acceptable solution-- after eating for two hours at Grandma's, driving home, and eating one of Mom's massive repasts--was to pray that my body would be there for me the day after.

In later years, joining the army and then the air force, I came to a major juncture. Fast food restaurants were slow in comparison to the force's dining halls. Fast eating was survivial. You grabbed what you could from the table onto your plate and stuffed it into your mouth. Sometimes I skipped the plate. Dinnertime was, in many cases, shorter than the time it takes for the Empire State Building elevator to climb three flights. Graduating from the air force provided me with a lifetime skill: eating as fast as I could, like there was no tomorrow.

Equipped with tremendous eating skills in terms of both velocity and quantity, I landed in the USA, where I was forced to evaluate myself and make some changes. The actions I took and the results I achieved will last me a lifetime. I came to this country almost fourteen years ago. I was 25 years old, had just left the Israeli Air Force, and was in peak physical condition due to the fact that I had been responsible for the pilots and officers' fitness conditioning.

Like most new immigrants, on my first day in the Big Apple I found myself eating my first Big Mac ever. I repeated this ingenious finding at least once a day, disputing with myself, which one is better—Burger King or McDonalds? Six months later, my 143-pound body had expanded to 178 pounds, which, for my 5'6" frame, was an astronomical amount. Yes, I had gained 35 pounds, but I still did not know which burger was better. At that time, I really felt as though I had betrayed my profession. How dare I teach and preach physiology and nutrition when I looked like an ad for a tire company?

Using the information that I would develop into the Anti-Diet program, I took action, and seven months later had returned to 143 pounds. Thirteen years later, I remain at this weight and have never dieted. I merely continue my normal lifestyle—a lifestyle that incorporates proper nutrition and adequate activity. By the way, I still do not know which is better, Burger King or McDonald's.

The *Anti-Diet* contains the before-and-after lifestyle stories of people like you and me— those who have faced the many problems associated with traditional diets. They ultimately discovered, adopted, and stayed with the healthiest way to lose weight: The Anti-Diet.

In this book I challenge the conventional diets, the commercial diets, and the costly weight loss programs. I present scientific evidence that reveals that *you really have to eat in order to lose.* However, you have to know how and what to eat. This is exactly where you will make the changes. Moderate changes, small changes; but we have to take what appears to be an unconventional approach, because conventional diets do not work.

The program in this book is not just a diet to get on and then fall off. It is not a misleading trick that will let you lose weight and then gain it back. It's a healthy way of eating, a happier way of living—a healthy lifestyle. It will create for you a sense of abundance rather than deprivation.

Not a day passes without a new finding about food and it's effect on us. However, we the people keep getting fatter every day. There is only one explanation for this disturbing phenomenon. DIETS DO NOT WORK! It's time to understand that the body is an intricate physiological machine with its own rules and regulations for weight loss and weight gain. A good working knowledge of nutrition and physiology is a great combination for a healthy lifestyle—and the greatest enemy of diets. Therefore, understand that this book is not a diet book. Diets never work, and this book will simplify the physiological reasons for it.

When I look in my dictionary, I find the definition of "diet" as "sort of food usually eaten by a person, community, etc." A second definition describes diet as "a sort of food to which a person is limited for medical reasons." There's no mention of restriction, deprivation, or hunger. I interpret the definition of diet as simply a way of eating. Instead of a diet, I choose to refer to this concept as proper nutrition, or correct and proper eating habits.

With respect to the Anti-Diet goal to educate you about a healthy lifestyle that will last you a lifetime, here is a letter I received from one of my clients, Tyrone, the sales director of a large moving company:

I joined your program and within eight weeks had not only made a major impact in weight and general conditioning, but acquired direct health benefits in respect to a lung condition and an operation-affected muscle area. By learning about food and its roles in my life from a nutritional and physiological standpoint, I was able to realign old eating habits. More importantly, I could make this adjustment with a positive attitude.

Like Tyrone, many people found education responsible for changing their lives, attitudes, lifestyles, and health. They stopped dieting. All they did was change their eating habits, become more active, and educate themselves about how to exercise. They learned how to read labels, how to eat in restaurants, how to deal with regular daily events as well as special occasions, such as weddings, bar mitzvahs etc.

One of the major changes I made in my life was related to my perception of my jogging activity. Back home, three kilometers of jogging (1.9 miles) was too far not to use a car. Today, a 4- to 5-mile (6 to 8 kilometers) is the minimum for my workout. I will never forget the visit to Israel, two years after I moved to the USA, where, after jogging for 23 minutes one morning, I found myself at the doorstep of my Dad's office, just beginning to sweat. Suddenly, my perception of distance changed, and even my country became smaller. Just a few years earlier, jogging to my Dad's office would been a major decision. But on that day it was a round-trip workout. It's all in the mind!

When Joe, appearing to be in his late sixties, first came to my office, he seemed very tired and worn out. As he described his health problems, his breathlessness and great effort in speaking spoke volumes of his condition. The following is an excerpt from a letter Joe wrote a few weeks after he graduated from my program:

I'm 60 years old and for the past ten years I've been suffering with a chronic condition diagnosed as COPD [Chronic Obstructive Pulmonary Disease]. This, combined with my over weight and sporadic exercise program left me out of breath most of the time. After six weeks [in Anti-Diet program] I've lost 18 pounds and am feeling much more physically fit and breathing better than I have in many years. Mickey has set some realistic goals for me and is giving me the knowledge and encouragement to move towards my goals.

When Paul, a former county attorney, came into my office, he knew exactly what he wanted. *"I want my energy level back; I only need to lose 15 pounds, but more importantly, I'd like to tone my muscles and lose my fat. I need to reduce my borderline high blood pressure, and I believe in reaching these goals, my resting blood pressure will return to normal. However, I have one condition to this whole deal. No one, but no one will take my evening dry martini away from me."* Paul the attorney kept his evening dry martini, closed an old chapter on his lifestyle, reached his goals, and never dieted again.

Janet came to my office suffering from Chronic Fatigue Syndrome, a debilitating condition that had forced her to quit her job and drained her of energy and hope. That day Janet began a life-changing transition to new eating and exercise habits based on the Anti-Diet regimen outlined in this book. She has never turned back.

I met Rob, the dean of a graduate school, in the health club where he worked out. Ready to make some changes in his life after the New Year's holiday, he came to my office and related a medical history of stress from a high pressure job, overweight, high blood pressure, high cholesterol, and excessively poor eating habits. Overwhelmed by his situation, Rob knew he had to augment his doctorate-level education with some straight, hard facts on nutrition. *"I want my energy back, I cannot afford to continue like this. I need to lose weight and I must eat better, not to mention the blood pressure,"* he said. *"The stress and the pressure at work do not help. I need a good exercise program to relieve those,"* he continued. Since that day, our well-educated dean has earned high marks in successfully implementing the Anti-Diet program into his life.

For Arnold, a master plumber, "sick days" had never been part of his vocabulary. Slightly overweight, extremely stressed out from the long hours and long daily commute that had become his routine for the past eighteen years, Arnold landed in the hospital with mild chest pain. Although he was released after tests showed he had not experienced a heart attack, the pain never left his body. A few months later, Arnold was readmitted into the hospital with endocarditis, which attacks the mitral valve

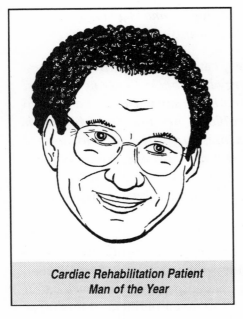

Cardiac Rehabilitation Patient
Man of the Year

in the heart. He underwent open heart surgery and mitral-valve replacement. As a cardiac patient, Arnie made the decision to ward off further health problems through the learning process of the Anti-Diet. And I became the happiest person on earth that day, because Arnold is my father-in-law.

Before meeting with me, Mardi had been to many doctors, dieticians, and even hospitals in an effort to overcome his chronic overweight problem. After putting the Anti-Diet program into effect, his life changed in ways that he had never imagined possible:

Mickey, you have given me my life back. Without your help in both nutrition and exercise, I was headed for disaster. I never diet and still lose weight on your program. Moreover, I eat the foods that I enjoy six times a day. You have given me an active lifestyle filled with education about nutrition and exercise that will be with me for the rest of my life.

Mardi armed himself with education about nutrition and exercise, and his lesson will be your lesson. It will be a lesson of health, of physiologically and psychologically, one of wealth.

Since 1987, I have treated over 4,700 clients like Tyrone, Joe, Paul, Janet, Rob, Arnold, and Mardi on my program. Each came to me with a desperate need to end the yo-yo diet syndrome or to improve a wide variety of health problems. And each graduated from my program with a priceless degree in proper nutrition.

Chapter One:

DIETS—THE WRONG SOLUTION

We are a Nation of diet-obsessed people. We gradually accumulate weight between the ages of 20 and 50, adding one to two pounds a year. Then one day we wake up to find ourselves carrying around 20 to 60 pounds of excess fat. We realize that we don't look good, don't feel good, and that the excess fat is likely to shorten our lives. So we resolve to go on a diet.

Between the ages of 30 and 60, many people lose over 1,500 to 2,000 pounds on various diets. During this period of time we "own" 17 health clubs, visit tens of thousands of diet institutes, and start uncounted numbers of diet programs. We successfully lose weight, but the weight always comes back, and in many instances surpasses the previous weight. Each diet provides us with a maintenance program that we follow for maybe 12 hours.

Why *Not* Diet?

Consider the following 1988 statistic: Since 1920, there have been 26,000 diets published in the United States. Twenty-six thousand different types of diets! That same year, 1988, The American Heart Association published a survey indicating that 95 to 98 percent of those starting a new diet will re-gain the weight within the first two to five years and in many cases will gain even more weight than they lost.

A similar study also published in 1988, indicates that the American diet industry had sales of $19 billion in that year alone. The following year the figure increased to $21 billion. Moreover, the amazing fact of this study was that $20 billion of the $21 billion in the second year was spent by the same people who spent the $19 billion the previous year!

You cannot win at weight loss by dieting.

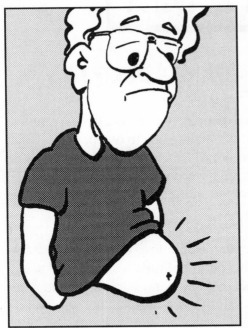

It is medically and physiologically impossible to lose 3 pounds of fat, not water, from the body in one week, not to mention the 5 pounds that some commercial diets advertise. If only 1 percent of the published diets delivered what they promise, we would all be slim and trim by now and you would not be reading this book. If diets work, why are we fatter than ever? Why are our children 100 percent fatter than their parents were when they were children in the 1960s?

We must be honest with ourselves. Look around, at the mall, in the supermarket, at work; look at our friends, our families, the strangers in the streets. WE ARE FAT! There is enough fat around us to feed one-third of the world!

It should be obvious that when twenty new diets are published every day, each one claiming to be perfect, something fishy is going on. The only reason for the continual popularity and proliferation of fad diets is that they FAIL! They all fail at making any permanent changes in people's eating habits. We Americans are currently eating fewer calories then we did in 1900, yet more of us are overweight than ever before. Why? The reason is that there is no diet now, nor will there ever, that the problem of being overweight.

Even worse than failing at weight loss, evidence suggests that traditional diets cause a wide variety of health problems. There is a strong tendency to regain weight, with as much as two-thirds of the weight lost regained within one year after completing a program—and almost *all* by five years. Only about 3 percent of those who take off weight keep it off for at least five years.

Worse than this, the yo-yo syndrome of dieting—losing some weight, then gaining it back—may be more harmful to your health than not going on a diet in the first place. This pattern/pathway is very familiar to just about anyone who has gone on a diet.

What Traditional Diets Have Proven to Deliver

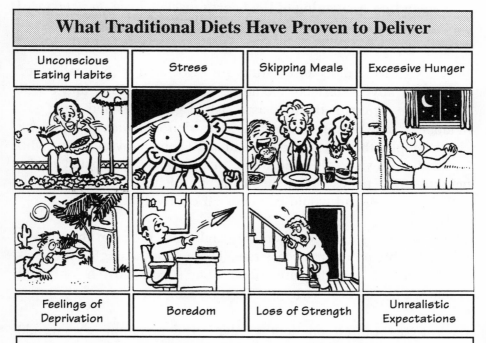

Unconscious Eating Habits	Stress	Skipping Meals	Excessive Hunger
Feelings of Deprivation	Boredom	Loss of Strength	Unrealistic Expectations

- **Unconscious eating habits** (*I'd rather be conscious when I decide what to put in my mouth.*)
- **Feelings of deprivation** (*It is scandalous to feel deprived in such a food-rich country.*)
- **Stress** (*Daily commuting stress is enough for me.*)
- **Boredom** (*With 12,000 food items in the supermarket, I can find lots of fun.*)
- **Meal skipping** (*Eat; skip rope not meals.*)
- **Low self-esteem and lack of self-trust and faith** (*Don't let them blame it on you. Stop participating in those diets, and start building your faith in what you are doing.*)
- **Excessive hunger** (*Why? Just eat, but don't forget to keep skipping rope.*)

(continued)

3

> • **Unrealistic expectations** (*Be honest with yourself, and your dreams will become reality.*)
> • **Loss of strength, motivation, energy, muscle mass, including weakening of the heart muscle** (*Given these factors you are on the road to GAIN, GAIN, and GAIN.*)

Very low-calorie diets and fasting are associated with a variety of short-term adverse effects including fatigue, hair loss, and dizziness. More serious is the increased risk of gallstones and acute gall bladder disease during severe caloric restriction. At least half of the obese people (those who are more than 30 percent overweight) who try to diet down to their desirable or "ideal" weight listed in the height/weight tables suffer medically, physically, and psychologically as a result and would be better off overweight.

There is not a single commercial weight loss program that makes data available on their success rate. There is not a single bit of scientific evidence that they are effective and successful. The only fact is that we are FAT! So why are we following them?

Each time you go on another diet of deprivation, the weight becomes more difficult to lose. So you become even more discouraged. This discouragement often leads to eating even more, causing more depression, then more overeating in a crazy vicious cycle. Eventually, you blame yourself for being destined to be fat, overweight, obese, or for having lack of willpower—all of which lower your self-esteem and diminish your ego.

The Anti-Diet: How to Eat, Lose, and Live

What you need is scientifically based information that will enable you to make more successful choices in your eating habits and your lifestyle. But you must make these changes yourself. No one wants to accept this. It is the hardest and the longest route. We'd rather take a shortcut, that is, If one quick-fix diet doesn't work, we can just try a different one. But changing your lifestyle to an active one and changing your eating habits to smart, efficient ones are the keys to overcoming the real reason for being overweight: lack of or slow metabolism.

Most diets that require you to deprive yourself of food by restricting calories may result in your feeling hungry and may actually cause your metabolism to slow down. (I will talk about metabolism in detail in the next chapter). Some diets may even cause medical problems; this is especially true of the high protein diets that are very popular today. They recommend that you increase consumption of meats and eggs, and that you reduce dietary carbohydrates. This can increase the risk of heart disease, stroke, kidney disease, and many other health problems.

Rapid weight loss is primarily due to losing water, but water and weight are just as rapidly regained. According to conventional weight loss commercial diets, learning gastronomy or becoming a CPA may help you lose weight. You lose weight on such diets by counting calories, carefully keeping track of everything you consume, and depriving yourself by limiting the amount of food you eat. The packaged diet foods usually do not taste very good, and you eventually grow tired of this type of complexity and hunger. You abandon the diet and re-gain the weight you lost and sometimes even more.

Despite that frustration, about one-half of American women and one-fourth of American men are currently trying to lose weight, with another one-fourth of each group trying to maintain the weight. One out of three females (ages 11 to 18) is on a diet to lose weight. Diets do not attack the fundamental problem in an overweight person. At the beginning of a cycle, losing weight is clearly not the problem for the overweight person. In fact, most overweight people make a profession of losing weight. The problem for them is gaining weight. For some of them, this is caused by eating amounts of food that you or I might have a hard time digesting. However, many of them do not overeat. They eat less than you or I without losing. They gain weight. Many of them used to lose weight, but no more. Now nothing works for them.

This strange phenomenon—of eating less yet gaining more—raises many questions. Why is it that my friend can easily lose weight and I cannot? Why is it that my spouse can eat twice as much as I eat and never gain? Why is it that even when I starve myself, I don't lose weight? Why is it that as soon as I go on a diet, I am totally starving and cannot stop thinking about food?

Recent scientific research in the past decade has begun to uncover the physiological basis of these problems. Certain changes that occur in the body on a low caloric diet and a low activity lifestyle make it progressively harder to lose weight and to keep it off. It is not simply a question of inadequate caloric intake or output, specific diets or a person's willpower.

By going on a diet, you are actually making it harder for your body to lose weight. Joe, Rob, Janet, Arnie, and Mardi were all facing the same problem prior to their introduction to the Anti-Diet: LOW METABOLISM.

What is the difference between the hungry slim person and the hungry fat person? The difference is that one eats and the other fights it. Usually the thin person is the one who eats. Why? To engage the fat-burning process, you must fire up your metabolism with the right nutrients and activity. The last thing that will remedy a low metabolism is restricting your energy input with a low-calorie diet. And the only thing that will cause effective weight loss is increasing your metabolism.

Like many people we know, Janet started aerobics with various weight loss programs in her mid-twenties. She just wanted to lose a few pounds that suddenly became attached to her during her first years of college. A commercial diet institution helped Janet lose a few pounds very quickly; she soon looked great and was ready for the swimming season. However, the diet institution failed to tell Janet that the low-calorie diet, which she followed 110 percent, would decrease her metabolism.

Two years later, graduating from college, Janet found herself endorsing a check to a second diet institution. This time she tried a starvation diet. Once again she lost the required amount, ready to beam at the beach. And once again, not knowing the physiological effects of diets and metabolism, the diet created a larger decrease in her metabolism level.

When I met Janet she had just given up on the $800 she had invested in a third weight loss program. She was without hope. Ten years after her initial diet, she was 35 pounds overweight with no muscle tone and a very high percentage of body fat. Janet had no energy and suffered from Chronic Fatigue Syndrome. Janet's metabolism was shot down.

Another client also came to me after many years of unsuccessful dieting. She had tried the commercial programs, the fad diets on the bestseller lists, the ritzy health clubs, the celebrity videos. At age 38, twenty years after her first diet, she was $10,000.00 poorer and 70 pounds heavier. Meanwhile, the diet institute's owners, who had profited financially from my client's fees and from many others, were golfing in the Caribbean!

What these clients and many others learned is that there is no diet now—and there will never be a diet—that cures an overweight problem. Diets do not attack the fundamental problem of the fat person. In the next chapter, you will discover the real answer.

Chapter Two:

METABOLISM

Our main goal in the battle to lose weight is to increase metabolism. This is accomplished in two ways: proper nutrition (or proper eating habits) and increased activity.

Some people find it difficult to believe that something as fundamental as metabolism can be changed. But one of the most exciting facts about our physiology is that, yes, various factors can change our metabolism. In most cases, we have the ability to raise it or to diminish it.

Arnie, Rob, and the others adopted the Anti-Diet program, which utilizes the thermogenic effects of food and exercise, correct eating habits, proper food content and timing, an active lifestyle, and a regular exercise program. All these factors made the necessary changes in our friends' metabolisms.

There are three main factors in increasing metabolism through nutrition, or proper eating habits: first, through the thermogenic effect of food (TEF); second, inhibiting the body's self-defense mechanism against starvation; and third, utilizing the thermogenic effect of food content. In other words, YOU MUST EAT. I just gave you a permit for life—EAT!

We know that you gain weight when there is an imbalance between energy intake, caloric intake, and energy output, based on the amount of your activity throughout the day. This is true, but it's not the whole truth. There are more fundamental questions to be answered. Are all calories alike? What affects the rate at which we burn calories? The answers to these two questions will give us a little more information about metabolism, energy expenditure, and energy imbalance. Meanwhile, leave the recliner and the TV, burn the remote control, and follow your children outside to play. In other cases, attach the treadmill to generate energy for your TV, and walk on it during your favorite show. By the way, do not tie the dog to the treadmill.

Make It Burn! The Thermogenic Effect

What is the thermogenic effect of food? When you eat an apple, for example, you take a bite, you have to chew it, swallow it, digest it, break it down into the various nutrients, and finally store it within various pathways in the body. What an expenditure of energy! If you skip a meal or if you're not eating, you are missing this part of the body's expenditure of energy. A good example is the college life pattern for four years and even more. The schedule from hell, lack of money, partying till dawn, alcohol consumption to the brim, and meal skipping result in the average female student gaining fifteen pounds or more in the course of the four years.

Based on this, eating four to six times a day, as is recommended for a diabetic person, is one way to increase our metabolism. This is the opposite of starving or depriving ourselves of food. To manage food the body requires some energy expenditure. When you eat, many of your body's cells increase their activity. The gastrointestinal tract muscles which move the food along, speed up their rhythmic contractions, the cells that manufacture and secrete digestive juices begin their tasks. These cells and others need extra energy as they come alive to participate in the digestion, absorption, metabolism, and storage of food. In other words, it takes energy to get energy.

Our bodies burn up a certain number of calories simply by converting the protein, carbohydrates, and fats in our food to energy sources. This stimulation of cellular activity is the thermogenic effect of food that consumes approximately 10 percent of the total food energy intake. Understanding this factor will allow you to raise your DMR (Daily Metabolic Rate) just by eating correctly. You need to eat to increase your metabolism and to increase your caloric output. *You need to eat to lose.* Eating four to six times a day will increase metabolism by approximately 10 percent of your total caloric intake.

Your Body's Starvation Self-Defense System

When you deprive yourself of food, as in a commercial diet program, the size of your fat cells shrink, but the number of fat cells does not. As a result, in addition to feeling hungry and deprived, your body thinks you are starving—because you are. It tries to compensate for the reduced intake of food by slowing down how fast you can burn what there is. This is the body's self-defense mechanism against starvation.

If you reduce your food intake by 20 percent, your metabolism rate may slow down by approximately 10 to 20 percent. When your metabolism is lower you burn calories much more slowly. You reduce your caloric output expenditure. Because of the self-defense mechanism against starvation, your body tries to maintain your weight. Even when you go on a caloric restricted diet, as you start to lose weight, your body tries to compensate on the supply side by increasing your appetite to force you to eat more calories, and on the demand side by causing your metabolic rate to drop. This is the dreaded "plateau phenomenon" familiar to all of us. It really kills motivation; you continue to eat less, yet you weigh the same. You're not losing weight.

If you are on a traditional diet and consuming 800 calories a day, the self-preservation system will kick in and not allow your body to burn more than 800 calories per day. As soon as you increase your caloric intake again, say to 1,300 calories, your body is going to be stubborn and refuse to burn more than 800 calories. This is survival. Your body is is not convinced that the deprivation times are over, and it's not going to take any chances by throwing calories away. It's going to store those extra 500 calories you're feeding it.

Take the situation of our friend Janet, for example. Her eating habits were anything but correct. No consideration of timing or food content, no set amounts, and worse than that, skipping meals and eating 700–800 calories per day. And she had no weight loss. Janet created a major reduction in her caloric output—her metabolism—due to her starvation diet.

Let's assume that Janet ate 1,300 calories a day instead of 700 calories a day. The thermogenic effect of food in the higher caloric intake diet would have been approximately 130 calories a day, versus 70 calories a day in the lower caloric intake diet. That 60-calorie-a-day difference would have helped Lisa burn 21,900 calories more throughout the year. This difference of 21,900 calories is equal to about 6.25 pounds of fat. And all Janet had to do was eat more food, more often.

If we eat four to six times a day and take in over 1,000 calories a day, we will bypass the body's starvation self-defense mechanism. Therefore, starvation diets are out of the question. Skipping meals is out of the question too.

Metabolism and Food Content

The third way to increase metabolism through nutrition involves the thermogenic qualities of food content. When we eat different types of food, the thermogenic effects of each are different. Also, our capability of storing food and the cost of storing it is different, depending on the type of food we are eating.

First, for 1 gram of carbohydrate, we consume approximately 4 calories. For 1 gram of protein, we consume approximately the same 4 calories. For 1 gram of fat, we consume 9 calories. This should tell you one thing; if your diet is high in carbohydrates and protein, you could really eat double the amount of food for the same amount of calories from a diet high in fats. You could eat more frequently and have much more food in carbohydrates and protein and still consume fewer calories than you would if they came from fat.

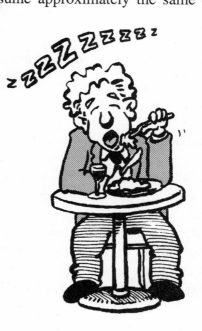

Also, when you eat fat you increase fatigue. The main reason for this is that fat is not an energy source. *Carbohydrates* are our main energy source. If your diet is low in carbohydrate you are fatigued and lethargic, which affects your metabolism and

Eating a high fat meal.

productivity. On the other hand, if your diet is high in carbohydrate and protein as opposed to fat, you can eat more and eat more frequently, become less hungry, and increase your energy source.

If you eat carbohydrates, there is a certain amount of energy that you need in order to be able to store that food, digest it, absorb it, etc. Approximately 23 percent of the total caloric intake from carbohydrates needs to be burned in order to store the rest. For example, if you eat 100 calories of carbohydrates, 23 percent, or 23 calories out of the 100 calories, will burn in the process of storing the rest. That means that only 77 calories out of the 100 are stored.

Eating a high carbohydrate meal

Similarly, 23 percent of calories that you eat from protein must burn in order to store the rest. On this basis, again using 100 calories of the nutrient of protein, you burn 23 calories to store 77 calories.

With fat there is a completely different story. You only need 3 percent for the thermogenic effect of fat. This means that you burn only 3 calories out of 100 calories of fat to store 97 calories of fat. Here is what happens: even if you eat fat in smaller amounts than you would carbohydrates or protein, you will be more fatigued and lethargic and have less energy. If you will eat less food, you will store a major portion of the calories. EAT LESS—STORE MORE.

Let's examine the utilization of carbohydrates, protein, and fat. What do you use carbohydrates for? Primarily for energy. You use carbohydrates throughout the day, 24 hours around the clock, to keep your entire system running. Protein is necessary for tissue repair and growth, and in very small amounts, for energy. You need protein around the clock, to keep rebuilding cells, converting protein to amino acids.

Why do you need fat? You need some for insulation and lubrication of the internal organs and for blood circulation. Much of the fat stored in the body is stored as adipose tissue. When do you use this type of fat? Primarily for energy, but energy that is burned specifically during cardiovascular exercise. Therefore, if you eat fat you eat less food and therefore become more lethargic and more hungry. It takes less to store it, so you store more calories, and the only way to get rid of it is to exercise cardiovascularly. No wonder most people in this country are more than 100 pounds overweight.

One of the main reasons for my gaining weight was the food content. Three times per day I ate a very high fat-content diet. If I had continued the same ingenious finding and had eaten daily at McDonalds/Burger King over the past decade, the weight scale in my office (350 pound limit) would not have been adequate for me a few years ago.

In summary, the thermogenic effect of food requires that you do the following for optimum use of energy from food:

To gain the optimum use of energy from food:

1. Eat four to six times per day: breakfast, morning snack, lunch, afternoon snack, dinner, night snack.
2. Reduce your fat intake, increase your carbohydrate intake, and eat sufficient protein. Eat 30 grams (or less) of fat per day.
3. Never skip meals. Eat a minimum of four times per day. Breakfast, morning snack, lunch, and dinner are a must. Afternoon and evening snacks are optional.

Increasing Metabolism Through Daily Activity

In your daily activity there are four ways to increase metabolism. One method is related more to your attitude towards activity in general. Three methods are related directly to exercise sessions and to whether or not you exercise. Our metabolic rate, or Daily Metabolic Rate (DMR), is built upon our Basal Metabolic Rate (BMR) and Exercise Metabolic Rate (EMR). These can vary drastically depending upon your actions and your decision to live an active lifestyle or a lazy one. There is no doubt about it—an active lifestyle can be the most powerful factor in increasing metabolism and therefore your caloric output throughout the day. Put Simply: STOP LOOKING FOR EXCUSES! Make a cognitive decision, and JUST DO IT! Become active.

Attitude

Prior to talking about exercise I'd like to talk about one way of raising your metabolism: your attitude toward activity. Daily Metabolic Rate is based much on what you do throughout the day.
Be honest, and ask yourself how often you:

- Walk rather than drive
- Take the stairs rather than the elevator or escalator
- Insist on finding the absolute closest parking space to the shops

The more activities you perform throughout the day, the more you walk, climb the stairs (the less you drive), the better you feel.

Another example of attitude affecting activity is when we mature, make more money, and start hiring others to do things for us, like raking leaves and mowing the lawn. These are things we'd be better off doing ourselves in the long run. This kind of activity will keep your metabolism higher throughout the day and keep your DMR higher. It will increase your caloric output expenditure and eventually it will help you with weight loss or with maintaining the current healthy weight you are happy with.

Therefore, the first way to increase your metabolism is through your attitude toward activity. The more you do, the more you lose. Adopting an exercise program will also deliver enormous medical benefits.

Exercise Sessions

Exercise lowers the risk factors for:

* Cardio-vascular disease
* Cancer
* Diabetes
* Osteoporosis
* Stress-related illnesses

Moreover, we now know that aerobic exercise has the most dramatic effect on our metabolic rate. It increases our caloric output during the time of the session while increasing our metabolism. Also, if you do cardiovascular exercise at the right level, at the right targeted heart rate, you are also increasing your body's capability to utilize fat for energy to contract your muscles. In other words, cardiovascular exercise gets rid of the fat from your body.

Exercise sessions five times a week for thirty to sixty minutes will increase your caloric output. This increase in caloric output will cause an increase in your DMR. However, merely looking at exercise in terms of burning a certain amount of calories in a certain period of time is an extremely limited perspective of the role of exercise activity in weight loss and weight control.

It is correct that if an average adult walks two miles he/she will burn approximately 100 calories per mile. It is also true that these 200 calories are equivalent to the one bagel the walker had for breakfast, and therefore it may not seem worth it to exercise. As I said before, this comparison brings us to a misconception about the role of exercise and activity in weight loss and weight control.

Post-Exercise Effects on Metabolism

There are two more effects of exercise on metabolism: Excess Post-Exercise Oxygen Consumption and long-term effect. Excess Post-Exercise Oxygen Consumption occurs when the Daily Metabolic Rate is increased drastically and remains elevated for as long as eight to twelve hours post-exercise. The engine is still ticking faster, requiring more energy, although you may be sitting on the lovesofa. Your body continues to burn more calories with an excessive amount of utilization of oxygen post-exercise. Let's look closely at what this means. If you exercise five times a week for about forty-five minutes at your targeted heart rate, there will be an increase in your metabolic rate post-exercise of anywhere from eight to twelve hours.

---

5 exercise sessions per week
x 10 extra hours of increased metabolic rate
= 50 hours of raised metabolism per week
30% of the week is spent with a higher, calorie-burning metabolism!

This benefit gives us a much wider perception of the value of exercise. It's not only how many fat calories we burn during the time of exercise—it's also what happens post-exercise for a third of our total weekly time.

Long-Term Effects of Exercise

At the time I decided to lose weight, I realized the profound effect of an almost daily activity regimen beyond the daily laundry. There is a tremendous effect of exercise over the long term. Your Basal Metabolic Rate is increased due to an elevated ratio of the over-all bone and muscular system to fat. When you lose weight by restricting the amount of food you eat, you lose muscle, fat tissue, and water. When you regain weight you regain proportionately more fat than you lost due to the fact that you have regained fat and water—but not muscle. You are not gaining muscle if you are not exercising at the time of weight gain. Therefore, you become fatter proportionately. You have much more fat

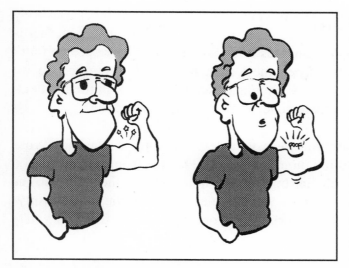

in your body compared to where you started in the first place. You have less muscle, therefore your bone density is also lower and your lean body mass is lower than what is was before. This interferes drastically with your metab-olism! You also get weaker because you have less muscle and less power.

What is the lean-body-mass-to-fat ratio? Very simple. One cell of muscle weighs much more than one cell of fat. One cell of bone weighs much more than one cell of fat. Lean body mass includes muscle, bones, and organ tissue. You increase your lean body mass by toning your muscles and increasing the weight of the muscles, which elevbates your bone density.

At the same time as you reduce body fat you are reducing the weight of the fat in the body. The higher your lean-body-mass-to-fat ratio, the higher your metabo-lism, and the more calories you have to burn in order to move that particular pound of muscle from one place to

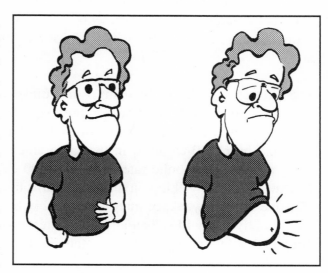

another place in space. Therefore, the goal is to have a higher lean body mass to increase your metabolism. Proof for this physiological fact is that for the fat people among us it is easier to stay fat or become fatter than to lose the fat and become leaner. Moreover, how often do we struggle to understand why thin/lean people can walk in the mall eating a whopping ice-cream cone, and maintain their weight?

Of course, the more you raise your lean body mass, the more your metabolism raises throughout the day for 24 hours, simply because you are carrying this particular body for 24 hours around the clock. So the effect of exercise is not only when you exercise for one hour or forty-five minutes. The effect goes far beyond the session itself as you're increasing your lean body mass and reducing your body fat.

Let's take an example of the lean-body-mass-to-fat ratio: a person who is 200 pounds has 40 percent body fat and 60 percent lean body mass. The 40 percent body fat represents 80 pounds of fat out of the 200 pounds of weight. The 60 percent lean body mass represents 120 pounds. For this particular person, 120/80 proves to be a ratio of 1.5 as the lean-body-mass-to-fat ratio.

The same person, a few years later, is down to 149 pounds, achieving a 51-pound weight loss. This person also reduced his body fat to 18 percent, which represents 27 pounds of the 149 pounds. His lean body mass is 82 percent, which represents 122 pounds out of the 149, indicating a ratio of 122/27, which is 4.5 for a ratio in lean body mass to fat.

The difference in the metabolism is incredible. The change in this person's lean-body-mass-to-fat ratio represents a *triple* amount of calories burned due to the increased metabolic rate. That means that if I just sit here and burn 100 calories, in the same amount of time, that person (with a higher metabolic rate) will burn 300 calories. Big difference! Just two miles of walking on the beach burns up 200 calories. If you do that five times a week, in three years you will change your lean body mass totally and will see an amazing difference in resting caloric output which affect postively daily metabolic rate.

The above also explains body composition and metabolism differences between genders. A man and a woman who weigh the same may find that the woman gains weight on exactly the same diet that allows the man to maintain his weight. By the same token, a man on the same type of diet treatment will lose more weight than a woman in the same amount of time. Why? Women have a lower metabolic rate than men because of the difference in body composition. Women generally have a much lower amount of lean body mass and a much higher percent of body fat than men.

With this knowledge in mind, exercise can have an effect. If one exercises regularly, it stimulates the synthesis of protein and growth of muscle. At the same time, it reduces body fat in order to produce energy for the working muscle. Thus, when you exercise, you are not only getting rid of unwanted fat; but you increase the amount of muscle in the body. This improves the ratio of muscle to fat, resulting in an increased metabolic rate and more energy expenditure. Muscle accounts for about 90 percent of the metabolic rate at rest, during exercise and post-exercise. If you lose muscle mass, you lose a metabolizing tool, and your need for calories diminishes. If you maintain inefficient eating habits, weight gain will be the end result.

To change his metabolic rate, Arnold the plumber was given a combination of correct eating habits with the needed nutrients for muscle tone, and an exercise program for body fat reduction and elevation of muscle tone. Through this program he changed his body composition ratio, or the lean-body-mass-to-fat ratio. At the same time, my intention was to strengthen Arnold's muscular system and his heart muscle because of his extensive history of cardiac problems. Arnold reduced his body fat weight by 25 percent and increased his lean body mass ratio. This elevated his BMR and DMR, important factors in maintaining his current weight.

Our second case, Rob, the college dean, had been living a sedentary lifestyle much like approximately 70 percent of the American population. I knew we would have to raise his metabolism with all of the ammunition we had. Making exercise part of his lifestyle was one of my main goals. Rob today is punching a clock in his local health club four mornings a week and providing himself with enough energy to condense three main jobs into one person's schedule. Furthermore, Rob's metabolism is at a level that allows him to consume normal amounts of food four to six times a day and maintain his 28-pound weight loss.

In conclusion, there are several ways to increase metabolism. Three through better eating habits, and four through exercise and activity level. Increase your daily activity, that is, increase your exercise sessions to three to five times per week. This type of exercise will increase your metabolism after exercise for up to ten hours a day. It will also change your lean-body-mass-to-fat ratio, increasing your metabolic rate throughout the day. At the same time, remember not to skip meals in order to increase your TEF (Thermogenic Effect of Food). Also, by eating all day you are defeating the self-defense mechanism against starvation, not allowing it to bring your metabolism down.

Lastly, your TEF calls for a higher carbohydrate diet with protein sufficient for your body's needs, and low fat intake will increase your metabolism by approximately 10 percent of your daily caloric intake.

The Five Golden Rules for Correct Eating Habits

The Anti-Diet program corrects eating habits based on food content and foods as applied to energy needed for the body. This involves foods and planning, food shopping, understanding food labels, eating food in restaurants, and more than anything else, foods and your personal lifestyle and culture.

People go to great lengths to acquire the skills and education necessary to have productive, enriching jobs and careers, to provide for their families, to make a comfortable home, to find personal fullfillment. But few take the time to learn the basic rules of nutrition and correct eating habits.

Rob was eating an enormous amount of food on the run. His fat intake was 45 percent of his total caloric intake per day. Janet did not eat at all—her diet averaged 700 calories a day with a 38 percent fat intake. Arnie ate whatever his wife put on the table. Whether it was three plates or four plates full, Arnie sat there and finished it all. Fried foods and a high fat intake were part of his daily intake. Paul, although better informed at the starting point, could not put all of the pieces of the puzzle together to implement correct eating habits as a way of life.

On the Anti-Diet program, Janet lost and maintained the loss of 36 pounds. Arnie lost 20 pounds, and has been enjoying his lighter and stronger body for the last three years. Thirty-five pounds lighter and four years later, Joe's doctor reduced his medication level and took him off the pulmonary patient list. Rob lost 28 pounds in order to eliminate the need for blood pressure medication. One year later he was taken off the medication after joining the education process at the core of the Anti-Diet.

Each of them ate correctly and still do. They have mastered the five golden rules for correct eating habits.

The Five Golden Rules for Correct Eating Habits

1. Cut down on fats and load up on carbohydrates. Make sure you consume 30 grams of fat or less per day, and enjoy complex carbohydrates such as pasta, potato, rice, corn, and bread.
2. Do not skip meals. We live only once: eat and do not deprive yourself.
3. Eat four to six meals a day. Breakfast, morning snack, lunch, and dinner are a must. Afternoon and evening snacks are optional. I'd go for the six!
4. Fill up your plate—to the rim! Enjoy it.
5. Never have a second serving. Don't be a pig. Six food intakes per day is more than enough. But, don't tell your mom I said so. Saying no to a second helping is denying the lifelong education by my Jewish mother, your Italian or Black mother, or any mother concerned about her child's growth. Saying yes to a second serving is accepting an invitation to fat city.

By following these rules you will feel less hungry, feel fuller most of the time, and your body will have enough energy to be very productive throughout the day.

Some physiological studies show other benefits from eating more frequently and in smaller portions. It's found to reduce blood insulin levels by about 25–30 percent. A typical high-fat, high-sugar diet will raise your blood sugar drastically, which will cause the release of more insulin into the blood. Many times it will regulate it to the other extreme and will cause your blood sugar to fall even lower. This is one of the reasons for the feeling of lethargy and fatigue. If you're eating four to six times throughout the day, you don't need to regulate your blood sugar level. The blood sugar stays at approximately the same level throughout the day, and therefore your energy level does not fluctuate.

Keeping insulin levels down also reduces the secretion of lipo-proteins lipase, an enzyme that increases the uptake of fat from the blood stream into our body tissue. By reducing this transfer of fat, we reduce the amount of fat being stored in the adipose tissue.

It has also been found that eating frequently reduces the cortisol level, which indicates a lesser amount of stress in our body. We've also found, in other studies, that increasing your eating and overeating many times is related to stress. Reduction in stress will help reduce the problems of overeating. Another effect of eating frequently is the reduction of blood cholesterol. If you succeed in reducing blood cholesterol, you also succeed in reducing the risk factors for heart disease and stroke.

In conclusion, eating four to six times a day reduces your fatigue; suppresses your hunger; gives you a full, satisfied feeling; and on top of all this gives you an incredible amount of energy. At the same time, it will cut down on the storage of fat in adipose tissue, reduce stress, and reduce risk factors for heart disease and stroke through reduction of cholesterol.

Chapter Four provides nutritional guidelines for the four to six meals you should consume each day. Chapter Four also discusses the adoption of healthy protein intake in this very low-fat regimen. There are three reasons for this, but one reason, I want to emphasize here, is that fat has over twice as many calories as protein or carbohydrate. Therefore, if you reduce fat consumption from 30 to 45 percent down to 10–20 percent of your total caloric intake, you can eat much more food throughout the day in carbohydrates and proteins and still not eat as many calories.

At the same time, the body easily converts dietary fat calories into body fat. In the previous discussion of fats, we found that the body takes only 3 percent of the total calories to convert the fat into stored fat in the body. This is compared to 23 percent of the calories that it takes to do the same for carbohydrates and protein. Therefore, if you eat much more fat, you will store many more calories— many more than if you eat carbohydrates and protein.

By keeping fat consumption low you receive two benefits. One, you will consume fewer calories. Second, you will be less likely to convert these calories into body fat because they are mostly carbohydrates and protein calories. You must remember: *If less fat goes in, you will be less fat!*

Chapter Three:

AN ACTIVE LIFESTYLE

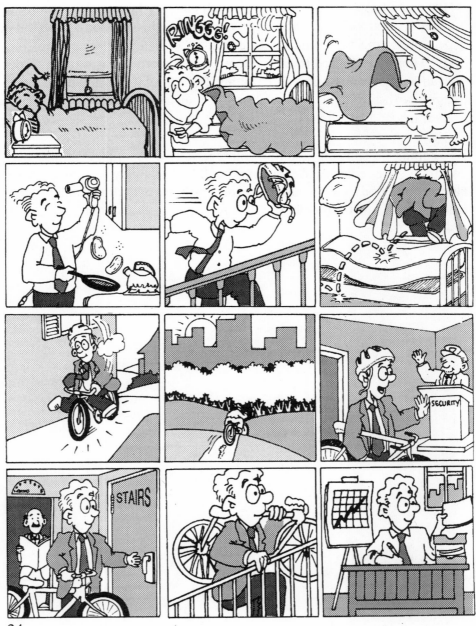

Evidence is rapidly accumulating to prove that exercise is the most effective way to control weight permanently. Exercise and an active lifestyle is our metabolizing machinery. Our bodies were simply not designed for the sedantary life or for eating sparingly. We are clearly meant to consume enough energy to support a good deal of physical activity. Nature never envisioned desk jobs, televisions, or automobiles when putting the human body together.

Americans are eating fewer calories now than in 1900, yet more of us are overweight than ever before. Why? A simple answer: less activity. We have greatly reduced the energy-consuming demands of work. Labor-saving devices are as common in the home as in the factory. Fewer people work on farms; more people engage in white collar jobs, sitting at desks in front of a computer all day long. For many people, physical exertion on the job is out of the question. And it is amazing to discover the lengths people will go to avoid the slightest bit of activity, in spite of the obvious health benefits.

The year I gained the weight—surprise, surprise—I did not do a thing when it came to activity or exercise. Standing by the street intersection, holding my hand up, and praying for an available taxi was my only out-door activity. Mouth motion in the fast chain restaurants was my constant indoor activity.

Joe had moderate to severe obstructive lung disease and at 55 years had convinced himself it was time to become active. With Chronic Fatigue Syndrome, Janet needed to stop to realize it was time to pick up energy. Arnie, our plumber, needed a mild heart attack and open heart surgery to convince him it was time to change his priorities and to become a more active and conditioned person. Another client, an attorney, required a mild heart attack, medication treatment, and a very concerned wife to convince him to change his lifestyle. He waited more than a year after the heart attack to begin exercising. He hasn't stopped since. Rob, the dean, increased his activity level only after his medical doctor notified him that he needed to take blood pressure medication until he lost weight.

An active lifestyle has been the answer for all these people. It is also the answer for low body fat, good muscle tone, higher metabolism, stress relief and many other benefits. Not engaging in such a lifestyle is a sin and an insult to your body. Eventually, the physical and emotional punishment will appear. However, starting to exercise and becoming active is still easier said than done. The anti-exercise movement is global and stronger than the American dollar, the Japanese yen, and the German mark collectively. My Dad used to remind me of the invention of the car in the current century, "so why jog?" With cancer and a heart condition, a suffering CEO of a marketing management company was perhaps convinced to check his mail four times a day, because the only other exercise he was willing to do was to abuse all of us humorously.

You must raise a few questions and honestly evaluate your daily activity and exercise level. How active are you? Do you have an active job or a desk job? Is your job sedentary or labor-intensive? Do you drive most of the day? How active are you at home? Do you come home and collapse with the newspaper in front of the TV, watch a few shows and go to sleep? Or do you help clean the house, play with the kids and take care of the garden? Do you exercise at all? If so; how much, how long, how many times a week? Is it aerobic/cardiovascular/weight training/strength program, tennis, skiing, or playing soccer once a week?

In order to evaluate your activity level and exercise habits, take a normal (or average) week within your lifestyle, and record all of your daily activities during the course of the week. You should be able to evaluate how active you really are. Be honest with yourself.

In the previous chapter, we talked about increasing your metabolism through regular daily activities, and about your attitude toward activity. You can increase your metabolism just by driving your car less, walking more, taking the stairs more often than using the elevator, etc. Also, it's time to engage in an exercise program. There are many books on the subject, and you can learn how to start safely and gradually. But the following pointers will not only help you create a simple exercise program, but also regulate your weight.

The first thing you must do prior to starting any exercise program, is to check out your medical condition with your physician. Remember, it is your responsibility to make sure that exercise is SAFE for you. Check with your physician or physiologist to see if you need any medication to control blood pressure, etc., and to determine if it is safe for you to begin.

To reduce the risk factors for heart disease, weight and fat loss, or for better cardio-vascular conditioning, an aerobic exercise program is recommended. An aerobic exercise program is the one that will increase caloric output and will increase the fat caloric output, which means you are burning fat. So for higher fat loss, as well as for the reduction of risk factors, cardiovascular is the recommended type of exercise. That means that the activity mode should be an aerobic activity—walking, jogging, cycling, etc.

Walking

Walking is one of the most highly recommended type of exercise. We were born to walk. So, get yourself a good pair of proper walking shoes, put them on your feet, and start walking. Walking will be the least expensive and the easiest way to begin exercising in a cardiovascular program.

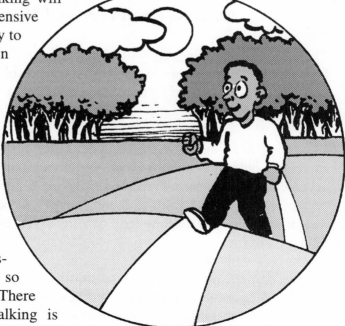

Of course, if you can afford to invest in cardiovascular equipment for your home, or join a health club and use the sophisticated machinery, so much the better. There is no excuse—walking is the ideal start. But remember, most health club newcomers quit within two to three months. That is an eight- to twelve-week commitment. Did you ever wonder how a 30,000 square-foot facility with limited cardio-vascular exercise machines can have over 2,000 members? Can you imagine what would have happened if even half of them showed up at any given time after work? Joining a health club is efficient and beneficial for some, but not for all. Most of the home exercise machines can produce results for many of us. However, in my experience with many of my clients, these machines over time become just another piece of dusty furniture or a major laundry hanging tool. For my towels and underwear, I prefer a laundry line rather than a $1,500.00 exercise machine. Your best bet is walking.

In order to begin walking for health, or in order to begin any exercise program, the first thing you need to do is to make the decision that there will be no excuses. You must make a decision to consider exercise a normal part of your lifestyle—as habitual as brushing your teeth in the morning. Remember, even four visits to the mailbox at the end of the driveway is better than sending the dog to pick up the mail and can be a key to your success.

Exercise Frequency and Duration

The recommended frequency of exercise is three to five times a week. Of course, the more you do, the better your results will be. I'd rather you begin your program by exercising three times a week, move on to four, and then advance to five.

Exercising five times a week, produces faster and superior results than exercising only three times a week. But do not push yourself to six and seven times a week for two reasons. First, the benefits that you gain will be temporary, for two to three months, until you burn out and give up. This is in contrast to the long-term benefits of exercising over an extended period of time.

The second reason not to exercise six to seven times per week is the danger of developing long-term injuries such as tendonitis, Achilles tendon problems, knee problems, hip joint problems, and lower-back

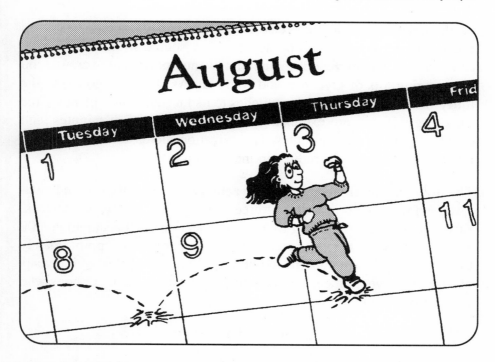

trouble. Giving yourself a break once and awhile is giving your body time to recuperate and to prepare itself for the next workout.

As for the duration, you must exercise over thirty minutes for each session. But if you are just starting your own exercise program, your goal is to work up to this amount. Start with five-, ten-, and twenty-minute exercise periods, building endurance slowly. Then continue to build yourself up to anywhere from thirty to sixty minutes. Eventually, you can work yourself up to forty-five to sixty minutes—the recommended duration of a good walking workout. As you build yourself up, the better (and stronger) you become. And the longer you exercise over thirty minutes, the more fat you burn.

Do not fall for the advertisement for certain exercise programs or machines that promise you the remarkable body of twenty-two-year-old male and female models. First of all, not only are younger than you, with better heredity than me or you, but they exericise a few hours a day, every day, and get paid for it. They could not build up such pictorial, sculptured bodies by exercising three times a week, twelve minutes a session.

At the beginning of any exercise session, your body is more likely to utilize more glycogen than fat as an energy source so that the muscle can contract. Therefore, during the first twenty minutes of exercise, you are utilizing lots of glycogen and some fat. As you keep going, to the thirty-minute point, the body switches to its fat source as a main source for energy. If you are exercising for thirty to forty-five minutes, and eventually up to sixty minutes, fat utilization increases, and therefore body fat and weight fat reduction increases too.

The duration and frequency of your activity is the most profound catalyst for fat reduction. Walking three miles a day, four times a week, fifty weeks a year (allowing two weeks vacation) will accumulate 600 miles of walking for the year. This is comparable to approximately twenty-three walk marathons in one year. In my short thirty-nine years of life, I have yet to meet anyone who has walked in 23 marathons who is fat or overweight.

Exercise Intensity

To gain the maximum benefits of exercise, you should exercise to the point of exerting a mild to moderate sweat and mild hyperventilation. Intense exercise, in many cases, should be prescribed by your family physician or by an exercise physiologist based on an exercise-graded stress test. If you do take a stress test and start walking on your own, the rules above still applies—exercise to a point where you feel just a mild to moderate sweat and mild hyperventilation. Remember, becoming a red, tomato face, green, or yellow, will not result in fat or weight reduction.

One way of determining how hard you can really push yourself is the "talking test." You want to be sure that you can talk to people who are exercising with you. Although it may be difficult to do during the early days of your program, you should be right on the borderline of being able to strike up a conversation. If you do have an exercise prescription from a physician or exercise physiologist, just stick to it and do not raise the levels on your own. Make sure that the professional people raise the levels of intensity for you so you will be exercising at a level based on your medical condition.

Exercise is one of the most important factors in increasing metabolism. It is an incredibly important factor in gaining the benefits discussed throughout this book. Exercise is also the main thing that helps you regulate weight loss or weight maintenance once you have achieved your ideal weight.

Make exercise a part of your life for the rest of your life. When starting an exercise program, begin slowly, gradually increasing the frequency, duration, and intensity. But use your common sense, or, in most cases, use your physician's advice. It is generally recommended that if you are over 35 years old and have not exercised for awhile, consult a physician first. And remember, walking is the easiest, most natural, and least expensive way of exercising.

Last note: If you do not like the word exercise and its associations (laziness, sweat, etc.), just call it activity (feeding the birds, or even sex), or anything else—as long as YOU DO IT.

Chapter Four:

CALORIES AND FATS: QUALITY VS. QUANTITY

Let's talk a little about calories. Each gram of carbohydrate, protein, or fat contains different amounts of calories that will change your caloric intake and therefore your weight gain or loss. One gram of carbohydrate equals approximately 4 calories. One gram of protein also equals approximately 4 calories. One gram of fat equals approximately 9 calories—double the amount of calories compared to carbohydrates or protein. Therefore, you run into the same conclusion: if you have less fat and more carbohydrates throughout the day you will end up with fewer total calories, many fewer fat calories, much less fat storage, and a much higher energy level.

For example, Beth and Laurie are 30-year-old twin sisters who weigh the same, are the same height, work at the same job and both walk 3 miles a day. Beth's caloric intake is 1,500 grams per day, while Laurie's caloric intake is 2,000 per day. Who will gain weight, Beth or Laurie? It's easy to assume that it would be Laurie, as she is eating 500 more calories per day than Beth. But in order for you to answer this question correctly, you need to know more. How many of the calories that each of two ladies eats per day are from fat?

Looking more carefully into their diets, we find that Beth has a caloric intake of 1,500 calories per day, which includes a 40 percent fat intake, or 600 calories. Laurie's caloric intake is 2,000 calories per day with only 20 percent fat intake, or 400 fat calories. The difference between the two is 200 calories per day. If they continue to at the same rate, and Laurie continues to eat the same for 17 days, Beth will have 3,500 more fat calories than Laurie, even though she is eating 500 calories less per day. Three-thousand five-hundred calories equals 1 pound of fat.

This means that every 17–18 days Beth will put 1 pound of fat on her body compared to Laurie. The conclusion: *It's not how many calories you are eating, it's how many calories of fat.* You have to remember that 9 calories of fat is 1 gram of fat. We have to cut down on fat consumption; bring it down to the minimum.

Animal Fats and Vegetable Fats

Fats can be divided into two major categories: animal fats and vegetable fats. Animal fats come from meat, poultry, fish, seafood, dairy products, and eggs. Vegetable fats come from oil, nuts, avocado, olives, seeds, margarine, etc.

Whether it's animal fats or vegetable fats, 1 gram of fat equals 9 calories. For the purpose of weight reduction and weight maintenance, the most important thing to know is that we have to cut down on fats in order to cut the total calories that come from fat. No wonder I gained over 35 pounds in no time following a daily habit of putting a cheeseburger and french fires into my mouth, consuming more than 30 grams of fat in one sitting.

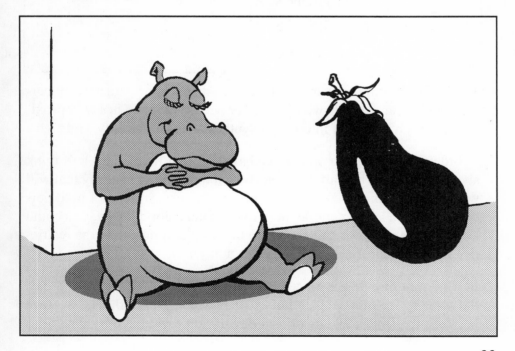

Animal Fats	**Vegetable Fats**
Meats:	nuts and seeds
veal •	avocado
beef •	margarine
pork •	oils
lamb •	dressings
venison •	olives
All other meat products •	Mayonnaise (no eggs)
Poultry:	
chicken •	
turkey •	
duck •	
Eggs	
Dairy products	
Fish and shellfish	
Mayonnaise	

The fat content in the average American's diet is approximately 40 percent, which far exceeds what we really need. The body needs approximately 10 grams of fat in order to synthesize essential fatty acids.

In order to do this, you do not need a 40 percent fat diet. So let's think about cutting this by half. Let's try to do it moderately in a way that will work for everyone reading this book. If you take, instead of a 40 percent fat diet, a 20 percent fat diet of your total caloric intake, you could also average out your caloric intake to a higher intake than the restrictive caloric diet (under 1,000 calories a day).

In a normal diet that averages between 1,200 to 1,500 calories a day, the total fat calorie intake should be between 240-300. The average between the two is 270 calories a day. If you divide 270 by 9 calories per gram, you find out that an active body can take care of 30 grams of fat a day and lose or control its weight. Therefore, 30 grams of fat per day—or less—is your number.

Daily Fat Requirements

For an adult weighing 168 lbs. = 10 fat grams , or 1/3 oz. of fat per day

Recommended range of fat intake for weight control:

10 to 30 grams of fat, or 1/3 to 1 oz. of fat per day

If you can eat fewer fat grams a day, excellent, but up to 30 grams of fat per day is OK. By the way, 30 grams equals 1.1 ounce. So, all we are talking about is 1.1 ounce of fat per day. All you have to learn is where the fat comes from. All you have to recognize is how many grams of fat are in a serving of the foods that you eat. Then monitor those foods so that you do not exceed 30 grams of fat per day, and you will be on the right track to losing weight.

Remember the Anti-Diet rule on fats: **Eat only 30 grams or less of fat per day.**

Dietary Guidelines for Proper Eating Habits

You have to remember that this is not a diet. This is just a guideline— you can deviate from it, you can eat anything that is exchangeable. For example, in the listing of breakfast foods that follows, you will see that you can eat a bagel or two slices of toast or an English muffin or a pita bread. You can take an apple or any type of fruit and exchange it accordingly to what you like and the type of food you will feel comfortable with as long as it is comparable to the guidelines I give you.

Again, it's not a diet. The types of food that I put together will provide you with two benefits. First, if you're not deviating from it, your caloric intake will be anywhere between 1,200–1,500 calories per day, which will create a deficit in your caloric intake. If you are also active, you will lose weight. Second, in any combination you take, as long as you follow the rules in the guide, you are not surpassing 30 grams of fat per day. As a matter of fact, in most cases you will be under 20 grams of fat per day.

Dietary Guidelines for Breakfast

- You **must** have breakfast. You cannot skip it.
- You must have your breakfast within the first three hours of your waking day.

Breakfast food choices: (pick one)

English muffin
Bagel
2 slices toast
Cereal with skim, 1% or 2% milk
Oatmeal with skim, 1% or 2% milk

My choice

Bagel
Marmalade
Orange juice
Coffee

Plus: (pick one)

1 piece of fruit or 1 glass of juice
1 to 2 eggs only once per week

Spreads for muffin, bagel or toast:
(A very thin layer, just to taste,
of one of the following):

Margarine
Butter
Marmalade
Jelly
Cheese
Cream cheese

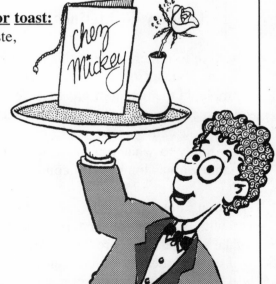

Dietary Guidelines for Lunch

- You must have lunch. Do not skip it.
- Eat lunch three to four hours after breakfast, preferably before 2:00 p.m.

<u>Lunch **food** choices:</u> (pick one)   <u>**My** choice:</u>

Tuna sandwich   Plate of rice
Chicken sandwich   Mixed vegetables
Turkey sandwich

Salad/Bread Combo #1: Tuna, chicken, or turkey on fresh green salad with vinegar and oil, lemon juice, or any low- or non-fat dressing Plus 1 to 2 slices of the bread of your choice

Salad/Bread Combo #2: Chef's salad without ham with vinegar and oil, lemon juice, or any low- or nonfat dressingPlus 1 to 2 slices of the bread of your choice

Salad/Bread Combo #3: Greek salad with small amount of Feta cheese and olive oil on the sidePlus 1 to 2 slices of the bread of your choice

Salad/Potato Combo: One of the salads listed above plus one baked potato with a very small amount of Sour cream and butter or salsa on the side

Soup/Salad Combo: Any type of soup except cream soups with one of the salads listed above Plus 1 slice of bread, unless the soup contains pasta or potato

Pasta/Vegetable Combo: Pasta Primavera with small amount of dressing or olive oil for taste Pasta with tomato sauce topped with a small amount of grated Parmesan or Romano cheese (top with cheese only if the pasta has been prepared without cheese, butter, or margarine)

(continued)

(continued from preceding page)

Rice/Vegetable Combo: Steamed vegetables mixed with rice blended with a touch of cooking or olive oil Chicken or seafood Chinese take-out food should ordered with absolutely NO MSG and NO SALT

Dietary Guidelines for Dinner

- Again, like breakfast and lunch, you must have dinner and can not skip it.

Dinner food choices:
(fill a large dinner plate
with one of the following)

Potato/Meat Combo:
Baked or mashed potato
Plus 3 to 5 ounces of chicken, turkey, or fish/seafood
No deep frying or butter

Rice/Meat Combo:
Rice of your choice prepared without butter
Plus 3 to 5 ounces of chicken, turkey, or fish/seafood
No deep frying or butter

Pasta/Vegetable/Meat Combo:
Pasta of your choice prepared without butter
Plus steamed vegetable or vegetable medley of your choice prepared without butter
Plus 3 to 5 ounces of chicken, turkey, or fish/seafood
No deep frying or butter

My choice:
Broiled chicken
Baked potato
Green peas

Lamb, Pork, or Beef. These meats may be taken in 3 to 5 ounce portions once every 10 days to replace the meats listed in the combinations above

IMPORTANT: *Meats may be broiled, barbecued, grilled or baked—but never fried or prepared with butter*

Dietary Guidelines for Between-Meal Snack and Night Snack

Morning Snack between Breakfast and Lunch : (pick one)

One piece of fruit: any kind *except* avocado
Bananas are an excellent choice with only 1 gram of fat.
One cup of grapes contain less than 1 gram of fat.

THIS SNACK IS IMPERATIVE—DO NOT SKIP IT!

I will never forget a story one of my female clients, the CEO of a major chemical company on Wall Street, told me. Her story made that snack even more imperative for her career. She was attending a very formal morning meeting in order to sign a big contract with a Japanese firm. Ice cubes were warm in comparison to the atmosphere in that conference room. By 10:30 a.m. there were no signs for completing the meeting. My client's digestion system signaled its need for a mid-morning snack with loud noises to the immediate audience. My dedicated CEO pulled an apple from her bag and without thinking twice took a loud, breaking crunch that triggered the biggest change of the meeting. The astonished Japanese delegation and American co-workers cracked soon after the first bite, laughed hysterically, and within twenty minutes the deal was done. "As long as I live, I will eat an apple for a mid-morning snack," was her remark folloiwng a 10.5 million dollar deal.

OPTIONAL Post-Lunch/Pre-Dinner Snack: (pick one)

One piece of fruit: any kind except avocado

Melba toast, crackers, pretzels, breadsticks, rice cakes, popocorn without butter, low- or nonfat yogurt

ENJOY THIS SNACK IF YOU ARE HUNGRY— IF NOT, SKIP IT!

OPTIONAL Post-Dinner/Night Snack

One piece of fruit: any kind except avocado, melba toast, crackers, pretzels, breadsticks, rice cakes, popocorn without butter, low- or nonfat yogurt.

ENJOY THIS SNACK IF YOU ARE HUNGRY—IF NOT, SKIP IT!

THE ANTI-DIET REQUIRED MEALS
YOU MUST NOT SKIP:

Breakfast
Morning Snack
Lunch
Dinner

ANTI-DIET OPTIONAL MEALS:

Post-Lunch/Pre Dinner Snack
Post-Dinner/Night Snack

Additional Rules for Proper Eating Habits:

- NEVER deep fry food
- NEVER cook or bake food with butter.
- NEVER take a second helping. If you're eating a baked potato, never take a second; if you're eating rice, never refill your plate; when eating pasta, never refill your bowl or plate. Keep eating small meals frequently — fill up the plate, finish it, and enjoy it; but never take a second serving.

The benefits of this type of eating are that you will not feel hungry or deprived. By not skipping meals you will keep your metabolism higher and receive many physiological benefits, including optimum energy. By eating more than 60–70 percent of your daily caloric intake before 2:00 p.m., you are less hungry and capable of burning these calories throughout the rest of the day. This is much more healthy than eating very little throughout the day and then eating a very heavy meal at dinnertime, which stays with you throughout the night.

Also, by following the Anti-Diet program you are not surpassing 1,500 calories per day, yet are eating an abundant amount of food rich in carbohydrates and protein, and very low fat. And, very importantly, you are getting no more than 30 grams of fat per day.

Chapter Five:

THE 300-FAT PIE: SAY GOODBYE TO CONVENTIONAL DIETS

One of my main goals in writing this book was to find a tool that would put a smile on Mom's face. Throughout my life I have faced creamy, rich, and tasty food that Mom made. How can you say no to a home-made chocolate cake that would put any wedding cake you've ever tasted to shame? And how many times can you say no to your Mom without creating the most profound enemy? These thoughts and many others on behalf of the good things in life, such as rich, creamy foods, brought me to the development of my best eating tool: THE 300-FAT PIE.

Now that you know how to eat well, I'd like to teach you a way of eating that will keep your fat down without making you feel that you are on a restricted caloric diet—or any diet at all. You will eat well and still be able to eat some of the things we all dream of eating, or would like to eat, or are eating anyway . . . such as a good dessert.

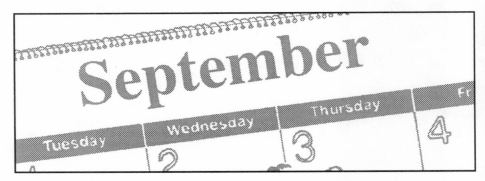

Let's take a 30-day month and divide it into three trimesters consisting of ten days each. If we allow ourselves on each day to eat 30 grams of fat or less, in ten days we have only consumed 300 grams of fat or less.

However, as you get better in recognizing fats and when to cut down on them, you can probably be fully satisfied with only 20 grams of fat or less per day. Based on a period of ten days, that means you are allowed an extra 100 grams of fat, just waiting to be taken in whatever dessert you'd like.

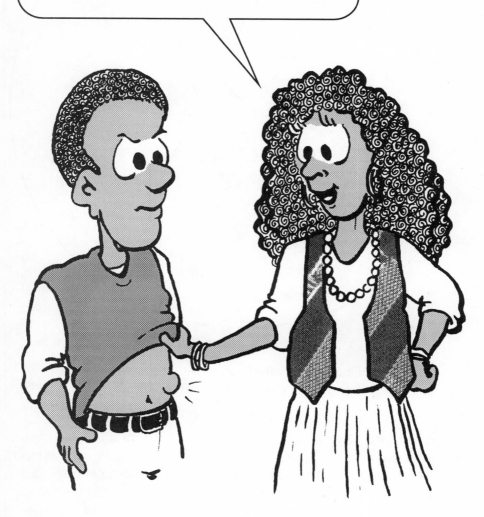

The 300-Fat Pie

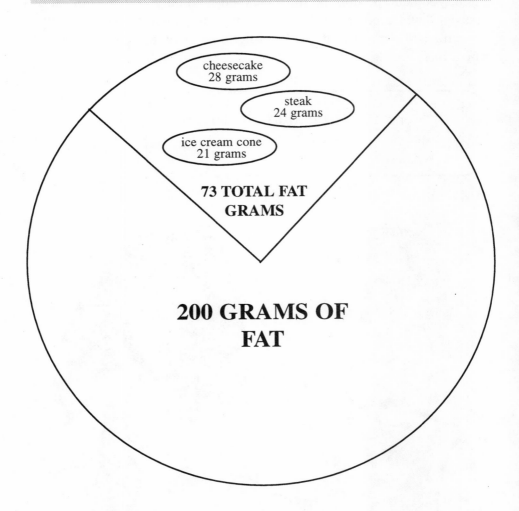

cheesecake
28 grams

steak
24 grams

ice cream cone
21 grams

**73 TOTAL FAT
GRAMS**

**200 GRAMS OF
FAT**

One-day fat allowance = 30 fat grams
Ten-day fat allowance = 300 fat grams

If you eat fewer than 20 grams of fat on each day of a ten-day cycle, you can allow yourself to eat products that are high in fat grams at least a couple of times in that ten-day cycle. This will create an average daily fat gram intake of fewer than 30 grams and will give you the feeling that you are not involved in a diet.

The 300-Fat Pie Applied to One Month

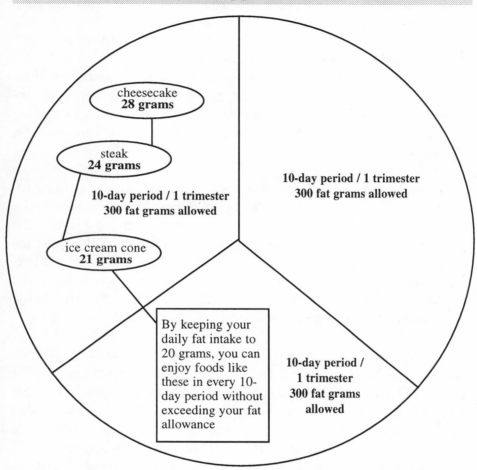

cheesecake
28 grams

steak
24 grams

**10-day period / 1 trimester
300 fat grams allowed**

ice cream cone
21 grams

**10-day period / 1 trimester
300 fat grams allowed**

By keeping your daily fat intake to 20 grams, you can enjoy foods like these in every 10-day period without exceeding your fat allowance

**10-day period /
1 trimester
300 fat grams
allowed**

The 300-Fat Pie eliminates one of the greatest problems shared by all the popular commerical diet programs: feeling deprived.

In some of these commercial diets, you are allowed only one meal and a liquid drink per day. You cannot eat what you want. You feel that although you are not eating, you are still not losing enough

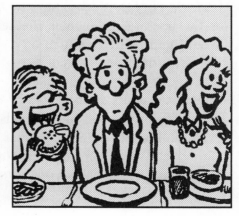

weight—or not losing any at all. You may be stuck on a plateau and simply cannot lose. You feel cheated. You feel you must explain to your friends or family that you are on a diet as soon as you enter a room full of cakes or cookies. You have to think about food all the time. All of this is related to conventional diets, and we need to demolish this.

You will not feel any of these things while you are enjoying the 300-Fat Pie. You will eat very well throughout the day—a high carbohydrate diet with enough protein for your body's needs—not exceeding 20 grams of fat per day. And you will have an extra 100 grams of fat allowed every ten days.

For example, let's assume that you would like to eat two slices of pizza, which will increase your fat intake by 18 grams. Or that you are in the mall, shopping around, when all of your friends move towards the Häagen Dazs counter and you'd like to have a scoop of chocolate ice cream in a cone. You realize that this is about 20 grams of fat. Or perhaps you're visiting your aunt who makes the best cheesecake in the world, or you're in a restaurant where they serve the ultimate marble cheesecake. This will give you another 18–24 grams of fat.

Now, two slices of pizza equals 18 grams of fat; a scoop of Häagen Dazs equals 20 grams of fat; and cheesecake equals approximately 24 grams of fat. If you take the sum of all three together you'll find that you just ate 62 grams of fat. A lot, no doubt about it; it is twice what you're allowed each day. But remember: in those ten days you only ate 200 grams of fat. Your core, your foundation low-fat regimen contained fewer than 20 grams of fat per day. Let's assume that every ten days—EVERY TEN DAYS you have two slices of pizza, a scoop of ice cream, and a slice of cake such as cheesecake. Would you still feel deprived? Would you feel like you're on a diet? Would you feel as though you were cheating?

The closer you stay to 20 grams of fat per day, the more you will be able to enjoy the rest of the foods that you usually are not allowed to even think about on conventional diets. Again, with normal, moderate eating habits you can eat a very low fat diet and at the same time enjoy chocolate mousse cake, your personal favorite dessert, the ice cream, the pizza, and occasionally a steak if you're still under the 30 grams of fat per day. Your body does not care where the fat comes from as long as it does not exceed 30 grams of fat or less on an average per day. Your body doesn't care, and you won't feel deprived.

Chapter Six:

PROTEIN

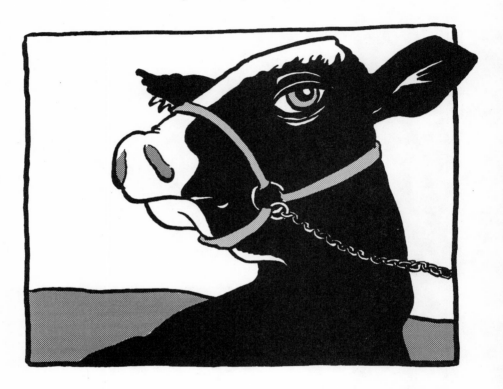

Many people still believe that a meal without meat is not a meal. For years we were trained to finish our meat off the plate and to skip anything else if we were not hungry. That need for protein has been as important for our survival as water and oxygen. We were told that protein is a major energy source. Football players and many other athletes were fed a 12- to 16-ounce steak the night prior to an athletic event. However, we were so deadly wrong! Protein provides essential functions to the body, such as tissue repair, muscle growth, and many biochemical functions throughout the body. Once in the body, protein converts into amino acids, which are used for those purposes. Protein is available in two sources: animal protein and vegetable protein.

Animal protein is very high in fat and, in most cases, very high in cholesterol. Vegetable protein comes from all kinds of beans, nuts (but these are high in fat), grains (most people are unaware that everything related to wheat, bread, etc is a protein source), rice, and pasta.

<u>Animal **Protein**</u>	<u>Vegetable **Protein**</u>
Meats:	
veal •	• nuts and seeds
beef •	• legumes
pork •	• all grain products—
lamb •	complex carbohydrates
venison •	• all wheat products—
All other meat products •	complex carbohydrates
Poultry:	
chicken •	
turkey •	
duck •	
Eggs	
Dairy products	
Fish and shellfish	

As an example of the nutritional differences between these two sources, let's compare one egg, (an animal protein source); and one bagel, (a vegetable protein source). Why were we told to eat eggs? Our mothers and grandmothers pushed us to eat eggs because of the protein they contain. One egg contains 80 calories, and one bagel contains 200 calories. The typical person will go with 80 calories

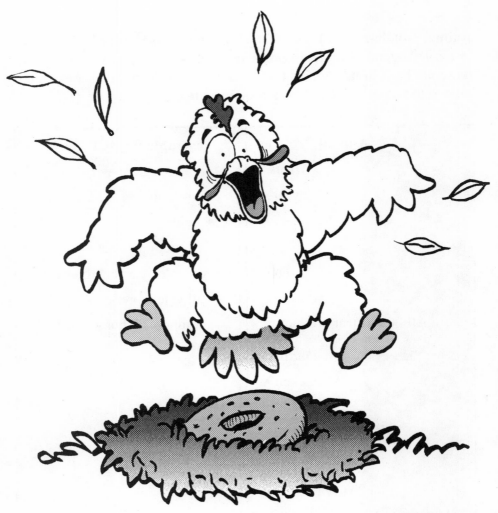

because he/she is eating 120 fewer calories, and therefore has more of a chance of losing weight. This is not correct, and the reason is very simple.

One average egg contains 5.5 grams of fat. This represents 50 calories of fat out of the total of 80 calories in the egg, or 60 percent. One bagel contains 2 grams of fat, which gives us 18 calories of fat—9 percent of the total 200 calories. Remember, we are eating the eggs because of the protein. However, one egg has 6 grams of protein, not to mention 274 milligrams of cholesterol. Your daily intake of cholesterol should not exceed 300 milligrams. One bagel has 7 grams of protein and 0 milligrams of cholesterol. What would you prefer to eat for breakfast? The egg—a protein source high in fat and cholesterol, or the bagel—a high energy source, low in fat, not a trace of cholesterol, and containing more protein than the egg?

How much protein do we really need? It's a myth that we need so much of it. It is essential to our body, but only in small amounts. And excessive amounts of protein will be converted quickly to fat. This means that if you eat too much protein from animal sources—meats and eggs—you will convert the excessive amount of protein to fat in the long run.

On the average, a person requires 0.8 gram of protein per kilogram of body weight per day. For ease of figuring, let's round this out to 1 gram per kilogram of body weight. For example, a person weighing 75 kilograms (168 pounds) will need 75 grams of protein per day. This is equal to approximately 2.6 ounces of protein. On the average, our bodies need between 2.5 to 3.5 ounces of protein per day.

Our Daily Protein Requirement = 2.5 to 3.5 Ounces

Four ounces of red meat contains 3 ounces of protein. Three ounces of poultry or fish contains 1.5 to 2 ounces of protein. This will provide approximately what you need from animal protein, and the rest will come from vegetable protein sources. Our bodies do not require a lot of protein! Don't worry about it; if you eat a high-carbohydrate diet with fish, chicken, or tuna, you are getting enough protein and you eliminate the process of converting protein into fat and storing it.

In addition to the fat gain, there are other hazards to a diet high in animal protein. It increases the risk of heart disease and stroke. It increases ketosis, kidney disease, gout and many other health problems. Weight loss due to a high protein diet will be a weight loss based on water loss, and as soon as you come off the diet, you will gain it back very quickly.

In the Anti-Diet program, you receive the amount of protein your body really needs and obtain more of it from vegetable sources than animal sources.

Chapter Seven:

CARBOHYDRATES: OUR MAIN ENERGY SOURCE

Carbohydrates are our main energy source; we need them just as our car needs fuel. Without them, we cannot function well. We find carbohydrates primarily in wheat products such as bread, grains, rice, potatoes, and pasta. Complex carbohydrates, starch, simple sugars, and fiber are all sugars. However, they can be divided into two major categories: complex carbohydrates and simple sugars.

Complex and Simple Carbohydrates

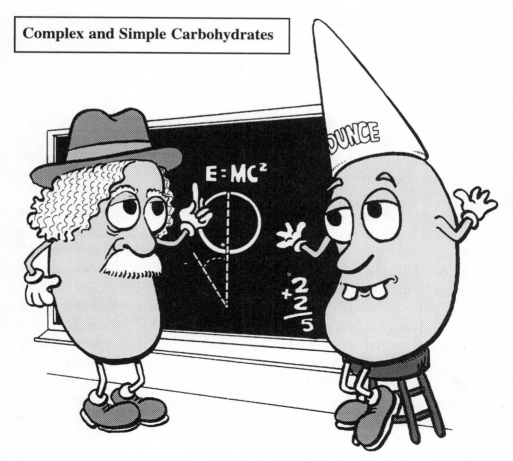

Complex and Simple Carbohydrates

Sources of Complex Carbohydrates

Wheat products:
>   breads
>   crackers
>   cereals
>   etc.

Grain products:
>   pasta products
>   rice products
>   corn and corn products

Potatoes

An important characteristic of carbohydrates is that our bodies cannot convert them to fat. You need to eat a tremendous amount of carbohydrates to convert some to fat; specifically, in excess of 4,000 calories a day. Remember, it is not bread that makes you get fat—it is the butter that you put on it. It is not the potato that gets you fat—it's what you put on it and how you cook it.

This reminds me of my Grandma, who almost had a heart attack when she woke up one morning four pounds heavier than the night before. Of course, the immediate blame fell on the pasta she had eaten the night before. What my Grandma did not know, and many still do not know today, is that complex carbohydrates are converted and stored as glycogen in the liver and in the muscles. However, through that conversion, the body stores glycogen with water in a ratio of one to three. When my grandma stored one pound of glycogen from the complex carbohydrates she ate the day before, she also stored and retained three pounds of water. The blame for the sharp increase on the scale was put on the pasta of the night before. What is important to remember is that these carbos won't convert to fat, and they are not the reason for the excess amounts of fat in our body.

One gram of carbohydrate equals 4 calories—it doesn't matter what type of carbohydrate we get it from. Complex carbohydrates come from wheat, bread, grains, rice, lentils, pasta, potato, corn, etc. The complex carbohydrates converted to glycogen and is stored within the liver and muscle tissues are the long-term, main energy source which we use on a regular basis. It takes a long time to convert complex carbohydrates to glycogen, and as it goes through this process it increases our fuel for various functions rather than storing energy as fat.

Simple carbohydrates are simple sugars—refined sugar, white or brown sugar, honey, and syrups like maple and corn syrup. We also find simple sugars in dairy and alcohol. Most of the various types of alcohol are 100 percent sugar. Sugar in dairy products is called lactose. Just as a tip, any word on an ingredient label that ends with "ose," such as lact*ose*, fruc-t*ose*, sucr*ose*, dextr*ose*, is identified as a simple sugar. Fruit is also a source of sugar, however, it is natural sugar if you are eating it directly from the source.

Sources of Simple Sugars:

white and brown refined sugar
honey
syrups
dairy products (Lactose)
alcohol
fruit (fructose—natural sugar, not processed)

Hazards of Simple Sugars

In the earlier chapters, we noted the many physiological and psychological benefits of a high-carbohydrate diet. Now, we will discuss the disadvantages of eating too much carbohydrate in it's simplest form—simple sugar.

If you frequently eat simple sugar in small amounts over a long period of time (i.e. one or two cookies eaten every twenty minutes for two to three hours) or if you eat a large amount in a short period of time (i.e.

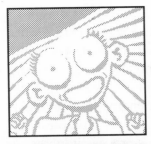

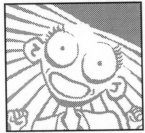

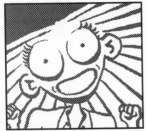

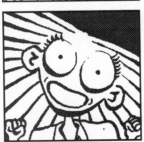

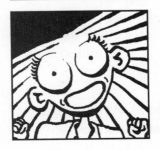

devouring a large portion of ice cream all at once) a few physiological processes kick in and have a great influence on our ability to lose weight. I believe that each one of us can fall into one or both of these simple sugar eating patterns at any given time in our lives. I recall demolishing a box of chocolate on the way home from the supermarket. A patient of mine used to inhale a box of Oreo cookies in his car on his way to my office. The picture of a Thanksgiving dessert table at my in-laws, with ten different pies and cakes, half of them eaten by the same family members within 45 minutes (adding over two cups of sweet coffee) is still giving me a sugar rush ten months later—and a need for a concrete plan on how to avoid the upcoming event two months from now.

First of all, these kinds of behavioral patterns cause an increase in simple sugar intake and an ultimate reduction of energy. As simple sugar intake increases, we get more fatigued and lethargic and, of course, have a reduction in productivity. With a reduction in productivity we see a reduction in caloric output and a decrease in metabolism, both of which increase fat storage from the calories of fat that we are eating.

Second, as your simple sugar intake increases the effect causes an increase in the blood glucose level. As the sugar level in the blood (blood glucose) goes up, you begin to utilize energy. If your sugar level is high, this is the first energy source that will be utilized. Simple sugar breaks down very fast and gives you immediate energy. If you are exercising the morning after a night of revelry (i.e. having a few beers, a slice of cake, and other sources of simple sugar) our blood glucose level will be high. Therefore, when you exercise you are utilizing blood sugar for energy.

If you are utilizing blood sugar for energy, you are not burning fat, and you are, therefore increasing fat storage.

Third, because of raised insulin level, there is an increase in the transport of fat molecules from the bloodstream to the cells in the tissue. Therefore, more fat cells are stored in the body.

Lastly, with the increase of insulin production we find that there is also a decrease in the release of Free Fatty Acids (FFA). These are the fat molecules that are utilized for energy. With the reduction of FFA release and an increase of fat molecules transported from the blood stream to the fat tissue, you're really getting a double whammy—storing more fat and reducing the ability to burn fat. So, yes, take a break and eat a Snickers bar in order to raise your energy level. But, in the long run you will pay dearly for it: your energy level after eating the candy bar will decrease sharply, while your body burns the sugar grams and stores the fat grams. No wonder you still feel tired after consuming of a candy bar! On top of that you put your weight maintenance in jeopardy.

As you can see, there is a tremendous disadvantage in high sugar intake, especially when we are talking about high SIMPLE sugar products. These will affect you drastically, causing you to increase your fat weight. Luckily, with the new labeling regulations, we are can see how much simple sugar of the total caloric count comes from carbohydrates in any given item. As a general rule, if the product has more than 30 percent of it's calories of carbohydrates coming from simple sugar, do not buy it. That way you will be secure that you are reducing your sugar intake to the minimum.

Follow the Anti-Diet rules on sugar:

Keep your simples sugars intake under 30% of total carbohydrate intake or under 20 grams of sugar per serving.

Keep your maximum sugar consumption to one serving in the a.m. hours and one serving in the p.m. hours.

Sugar and Artificial Sweeteners

The amount of sugar on the American table is an important concern. An average of 12 percent of the calories in the American diet comes from refined sweeteners. Roughly two-thirds of that total is sucrose, which comes from white sugar. The rest comes from high fructose corn syrup.

The highest source of our sugar intake comes from soft drinks, regular and diet. Both contain empty calories that provide no nutritional value at all. The enormous use of the dietary sugars and other caloric sweeteners is puzzling. The sugar concentrations in these products is so high that a very small amount should be enough to satisfy our taste buds. You jeapordize your health by using megadoses of these products on a daily basis.

There is a warning printed on the Sweet 'n Low packet: "Use of this product may be hazardous to your health. This product has been determined to cause cancer in laboratory animals." The effects of sugar substitute products may be even more harmful than we know. They also give people a further excuse to indulge in foods that are not good for them. The tongue can be fooled, but the body still wants its calories. Those who use these substitutes say to them-selves, now that I've eaten something without sugar, I can loosen up. People put artificial sweeteners in their coffee and then proceed to eat apple pie. We look forward to our diet drinks and share it with our favorite ice cream.

Per capita, sugar consumption has risen 14 percent since 1965, due to the increased use of sugar by the manufacturers of low fat and fat free products. The decrease in fat grams was replaced by the increase in sugar intake in these products. Rely on sugar in small amounts, but don't forget to exercise in moderation. When it comes to sugar, remember: not too much and not too often.

Chapter Eight:

LABELING

This chapter contains some of the most important information to make the Anti-Diet program work for you. If you buy food that is high in fat, high in cholesterol, and high in simple sugar, you are already losing the battle. Buying the right types of food and bringing home only those foods that can help you to lose and maintain your weight are the weapons that will provide a strategy for weight loss.

The new labeling regulations that went into effect in December 1993, help us identify good foods—their ingredients s well as their nutritional value. (See Appendix I for the entire regulation.) Learning to read food labels is an essential element for healthy eating habits. By the end of this chapter you will be reading food labels quickly and easily.

In 1990, a document from the United States Department of Commerce suggested that consumers demand food that provided convenience, quality, variety, and "health food" attributes. By that same year, an average of 12,000 food products had been introduced annually in supermarkets, more than double the number from the previous decade.

Obviously, healthful foods i.e., foods full of nutrients sell to today's consumer, and they have become an integral part of product development and marketing strategies. Common examples of this practice are so-called nutrient-content descriptives, such as "low-calorie," "fat-free," "no-cholesterol," "fiber-rich," "light," "organic," "fresh," and "natural." The term "lite" or "light" is used to imply fewer calories, reduced fat, lower sodium, improved texture/flavor/color, and even the amount of breading. Rarely is there any effort to provide balanced information about undesirable characteristics. For example, it may be literally truthful to label a food as containing "no cholesterol," but this may mislead consumers if it also contains a substantial amount of total fat and saturated fatty acids.

Buyer Beware! Label Deceptions and Nutritional Needs

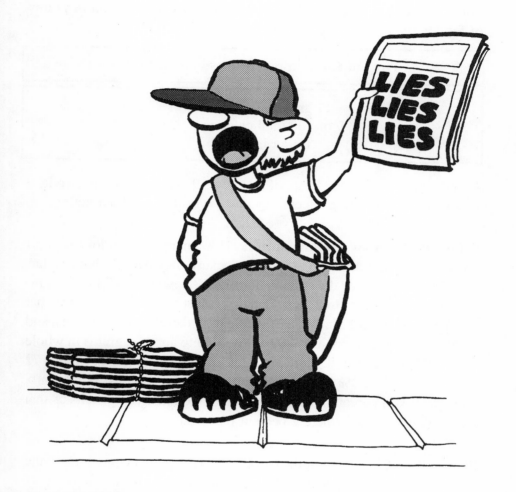

To determine the healthfulness of a product by its label, counting calories is not the most important task one has to perform. Moreover, comparing grams of fat to calories per serving from a product label is like comparing apples to oranges. Grams can not be compared to calories. They are two different measurements. However, 1 gram of fat equals 9 calories in any given situation. Therefore, to find out how many calories of fat per serving are in the product, you must multiply the grams of fat by 9 calories.

```
1 gram of fat = 9 calories
```

For example, 1 tablespoon of butter contains 100 calories and 11 grams of fat:

The Fat Content of 1 Tablespoon of Butter

11 grams of fat x 9 = 99
99 of 100 total calories = 99%
Butter is 99% fat!

Based on this fact, that 1 gram of fat equals 9 calories, let me introduce to you some interesting deceptions in the world of food marketing.

Whole milk versus 2% lowfat milk. How many people do you and I know who do not drink regular milk, because they believe that it is fattening; however, they do drink gallons of 2% lowfat milk? Let's examine more closely the strategies the dairy industry uses to make sure that we drink lots of milk. In 1 cup of whole milk there are 150 calories, and in 2% lowfat milk there are 120 calories. There are 8 fat grams in whole milk. In 2% lowfat milk there are 5 fat grams. Whole milk contains 72 fat calories, while 2% lowfat milk contains 45 fat calories. Whole milk represents a 48 percent fat intake. Our common knowledge tells us that 2% lowfat milk has a mere 2 percent fat intake.

SURPRISE! 2% lowfat milk represents 37.5 percent fat intake, and we're drinking it like water just to make sure that our fat intake is low—what a joke! In reality, the only difference between whole milk and 2% lowfat milk is 3 grams of fat per glass. It's your decision as to whether you want 8 grams or 5 grams of fat out of your 30 grams of fat allowed per day. However, the cholesterol level differs greatly between the two, with 33 milligrams in whole milk and 18 milligrams in 2% lowfat milk.

1 Cup Whole Milk		**1 Cup 2% Milk**
Calories	150	120
Fat grams	8	5
Fat intake	48%	37.5%

Butter versus margarine. The question asked of most nutritionists : Which is better, butter or margarine? The answer as far as fat content is concerned, will surprise you.

1 Tbsp. Butter		**1 Tbsp. Margarine**
Calories	100	100
Fat grams	11	11
Fat intake	99%	99%
	but	
Cholesterol	31 mg	0

Interesting! The ONLY difference between butter and margarine is the cholesterol. I believe that to most of us, butter is tastier. And if you do not have a cholesterol problem, I do not see a reason to avoid butter. Remember, moderation is the answer, and not deprivation. Whenever using butter, be aware of how many grams of fat per teaspoon/table-spoonful you are using, and calculate it into your 30-gram fat budget per day.

Take a look at the differences between margarine and imitation margarine products such as *"I Can't Believe It's Not Butter."*

	1 Tbsp. Margarine	1 Tbsp. Imitation Margarine
Calories	100	50
Fat grams	11	5
Fat intake	100%	90%
Cholesterol	0	0

The end result is that, yes, you have 6 grams less fat coming if you choose 1 tablespoon of the imitation margarine. But the ratio is still 90 percent of the total calories coming from fat! Again, don't look at the calories, look at the amount of grams of fat coming into your body, and make sure that it does not amount to over 30 grams of fat per day.

What about vegetable oil versus corn oil or olive oil? Oil is oil is oil! Labeling adjectives such as "no cholesterol," "all natural," and "light" are grossly misleading as to the nutritional value of these products. Any oil product gives your body a 100 percent shot of fat. Remember that, and use it in moderation.

If you do use oil, choose one that is the highest in mono-unsaturated fats, such as olive oil. The rate of heart attacks in the Mediterranean region, where olive oil is a staple, is lower than elsewhere in the Western world. The rate of breast and colon cancer is lower in Spain and Greece where olive oil is king. Therefore, if you do use oil in moderation, for better taste and health—choose olive oil.

Another very popular "light" product offered to consumers is a mayonnaise alternative:

	1 Tbsp. Mayonnaise	1 Tbsp. Light Mayonnaise
Calories	100	30
Fat grams	11	3
Fat intake	99%	90%

Again, while there is not a big difference in the fat intake ratio, there is a big difference in the fat grams. However, here is the problem. You're allowed 30 grams of fat per day, but many people eat astronomical amounts of low-fat mayonnaise, not realizing they re causing themselves harm. Moderation is the key. For the 9 percent fat intake difference, my choice would be to enjoy the real thing, useing just a little bit.

	1 Tbsp. French Dressing	**1 Tbsp. Low-Calorie French Dressing**
Calories	85	25
Fat grams	9	2
Fat intake	95%	72%

Of course, there is a big difference between 9 and 2 grams of fat, but consider how much of it you're using. Also, be aware that there is a high sugar content in any low-calorie or fat-free dressing.

Smart eating habits call for moderation, and I'd rather go for the real thing, using a smaller quantity. Drowning a salad in a 72 percent fat soup on a daily basis will have a drastic effect on the numbers on your scale and definitely forfeit any permit to eat a bit of chocolate.

Chocolate Without Cheating

A 1-ounce serving of chocolate has 145 calories, 9 grams of fat, 81 calories from fat, 6 milligrams cholesterol, and 23 milligrams sodium. That's lots of grams of fat, so if you eat chocolate, it has to be in moderation.

Chocolate has been put down by the cholesterol-conscious medical community because of its richness in saturated fatty acids. Sixty percent of the fat grams in chocolate are derived from saturated fatty acids, which is the major culprit in elevated plasma cholesterol levels—and a major contribution to coronary artery disease. All of this is scientifically correct; however, the saturated fatty acid found in chocolate is stearic acid. A major component of the fatty acids in chocolate is found in cocoa butter, and this does not raise blood cholesterol levels. This finding is not a license to sit down daily to a bar of chocolate but simply a permit to eat a moderate amount of chocolate products in the process of enjoying life.

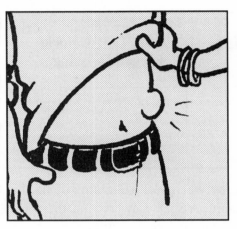

Remember, count the grams of fat, and if you decide to eat an ounce of chocolate, make sure you realize you are eating 9 of the 30 grams for your daily allowance of fat.

Sneaky Cereal Secrets

Cereal mysteries abound. Where's the fruit? Many cereal boxes show heaping bowls of fruit, yet it often turns out that there is not much fruit inside the box. Fruitful Bran, for example, contains 1.3 ounces of fruit—i.e., less than one cup. Consider adding your own fruit instead. Do not pay extra for it.

How do you spell "honey"? It could be W-I-F-E, or S-U-G-A-R. Honey is no more healthy than sugar, but because honey has a better image, cereal makers use it extensively in product names: Honey Nut Cheerios, Honey Smacks, Nut 'n Honey Crunch, etc. I prefer eating my sugar through a good imported swiss chocolate. Do not fall for this.

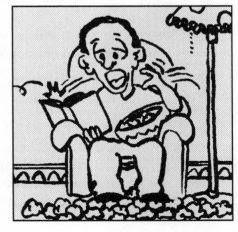

Fiber and crunch. Don't assume that a cereal is high in fiber just because the name sounds fibrous. Nut and Honey Crunch, Crispy

Wheat and Raisins, Rice Crispies, and Super Golden Crisps are low in fiber. And how about the sugar? Just because the name has been changed, the sugar level in several breakfast cereals has not been reduced. Sugar Pops is now Corn Pops, and Sugar Smacks is now just Smacks. But they're still high in sugar.

In conclusion, advertising and labeling information can help you select healthy foods. Note, for example, the use of a low-cholesterol proclamation on some brands of vegetable oil. This leads consumers to assume that other brands of vegetable oil contain cholesterol, when in fact no vegetable oil does. Cholesterol is found only in foods from animals.

There is a deceptive claim made with pure vegetable shortening that may be useful if you are restricted and you follow kosher diet laws. But if health is your main concern, you might be better off with butter and lard.

The two most saturated fats in the American diet are coconut oil and palm kernel oil, both vegetable fats. They can raise cholesterol levels and clog coronary arteries faster than any animal fats.

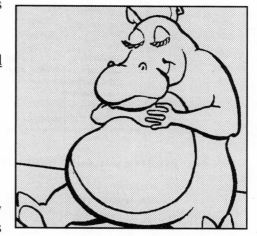

Products **High** **in** **Saturated** **Fats:**

• coffee creamer
• whipped cream
• imitation granola
• graham crackers

They are used in many processed food products because the oils are cheap, readily available, and have a long shelf life. Remember, do not trust what the label is trying to sell you. Some smart marketer designed that label.

```
┌─────────────────────────────────────────────┐
│  18% OF CALORIES FROM FAT                     │
├─────────────────────────────────────────────┤
```

Nutrition Facts

Serving Size 1 Bar (28g)
Servings Per Container 10

Amount Per Serving

Calories 110   Calories from Fat 20

	% Daily Value*
Total Fat 2g	**3%**
Saturated Fat 0.5g	**3%**
Cholesterol 0mg	**0%**
Sodium 100mg	**4%**
Total Carbohydrate 22g	**7%**
Dietary Fiber 1g	**4%**
Sugars 10g	
Protein 2g	

Iron	2%

Not a significant source of Vitamin A, Vitamin C, Calcium.
* Percent Daily Values are based on a 2,000 calorie diet.
Your daily values may be higher or lower depending on
your calorie needs:

		Calories:	2,000	2,500
Total Fat	Less than		65g	80g
Sat Fat	Less than		20g	25g
Cholesterol	Less than		300mg	300mg
Sodium	Less than		2,400mg	2,400mg
Total Carbohydrate			300g	375g
Dietary Fiber			25g	30g

Calories per gram:
Fat 9 • Carbohydrate 4 • Protein 4

The granola bar label above tells me two important things:

1)   I do not think that 2.0 grams of fat, taken in this small serving, is worth it;

2)   Sugars, at 10 grams, are higher than one-third of the total carbohydrates (21 total carbohydrates ÷ 3 = 7 grams). Sugars should not exceed 7 grams, therefore this supposedly healthy snack is not my best choice.

Nutrition Facts Serving size 1/2 oz. (14g) Servings Per Package 8 **Calories** 50 Fat Cal. 9 *Percent Daily Values (DV) are based on a 2,000 calorie diet.	Amount/serving	% DV*	Amount/serving	% DV*
	Total Fat 1g	**2%**	**Total Carb.** 11g	**4%**
	Sat.Fat 0g	**0%**	Fiber 1g	**4%**
	Cholest. 0mg	**0%**	Sugars 0g	
	Sodium 165mg	**7%**	**Protein** 1g	
	Vitamin A 0% • Vitamin C 8% • Calcium 0% • Iron 4%			

The snack label above (baked potato chips) delivers a different story: low fat, low sodium, and no sugar. Yes, some potato chips are good for us!

Remember, moderation is the key to healthy eating, and watching how many grams of fat you are taking in—you don't want to surpass 30 grams of fat per day.

Labeling and Food Shopping

When you look at food labeling, look for the breakdown given on the label. Do not fall for the deceptive headings, titles, or claims on the product labels. Here's what you need to know to make an informed decision as to whether you toss a product into your shopping cart or you leave it on the shelf.

Rule #1: Make sure that the serving size is the standard acceptable measurement; 1 ounce, 1 cup, 1 tablespoon, 1 slice, or 1 each. Make sure you recognize how many calories per serving are in the product.

Rule #2: If the product has more than 450 milligrams of sodium per serving—DO NOT BUY IT. Remember, sodium retains water and affects your weight loss. Also, for about one-third of the population in this country, sodium will increase blood pressure. High blood pressure is a major risk for stroke.

Rule #3:   The Fat Rule. Find out how many grams of fat are in each serving. Based on your daily 30-gram fat allowance, it is your decision whether to buy it or not.

Rule #4:   If simple sugar intake is larger that one-third of total carbohydrates — DO NOT BUY IT.

Rule #5:   If there is no breakdown of information on the product, which means no nutritional information—DO NOT BUY IT. This means that the product is high in either salt, fat, sugar, or all of the above. Do not buy the item if there is no nutritional information given on the label. Would you buy a car without knowing anything about it?

Rule #6:   Use your common sense. If you follow the rules listed above and use your common sense, you won't have the wrong type of food in your house.

Here's another tip for putting your new label expertise to work right away: pull out all of the food products you currently have in your home—from the pantry, refrigerator, freezer, and cupboards. Check them out to see if they meet the above rules. If they are too high in fat or sodium, attempt to return them to the store.

Each time you shop, choose only those products that meet your specifications. Using the following shortcuts, you will learn to make quick, smart decisions in no time.

Making Healthy Choices at a Glance

I want to teach you an elimination process. This process will allow you to choose a healthy product at the supermarket within seconds.

Check the product for a list of nutritional information. If it doesn't have any, just put it back on the shelf.

•If the product lists nutritional information, take a closer look. Check the amount of sodium milligrams per serving. If it's over 450 milligrams per serving, just put it back on the shelf and don't buy it!

•If over one-third of the product's total carbohydrate grams come from sugars, do not buy it. (Be aware! Most diet products, especially nonfat products, are loaded with sugars. The effect of sugars on the body's capability to get rid of fat is tremendous. Note: how many people who swear by the nonfat product as their major intake are fat or obese? Why, if we eat nonfat yogurt, do we not get rid of the fats? A nonfat product with a high sugar concentration is a marketing trap, not a weight loss tool.)

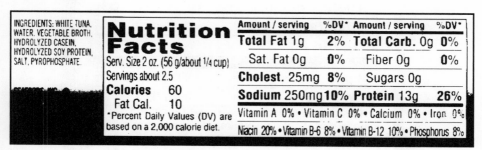

Note the serving size on this tuna label: 2 ounces. The nutritional facts on the label refer to a serving size that is less than one-third of the contents in the can. Also, at 250 milligrams, the sodium content is below the maximum 450 milligram rule. But that is for one-third of the can: If you eat the contents of the entire can, the sodium count zooms to 750+ milligrams. Too high! If you have water retention and/or problems with hypertension, make sure that the sodium count is low in every product you purchase.

CINNAMON GRAHAMS...
- ## No Cholesterol
- ## Low Saturated Fat

Nutrition Facts

Serving Size 5 crackers (32g)
Servings Per Container About 14

Amount Per Serving

Calories 140	Calories from Fat 25

	% Daily Value*
Total Fat 3g	**4%**
Saturated Fat 0.5g	**2%**
Polyunsaturated Fat 0g	
Monounsaturated Fat 1g	
Cholesterol 0mg	**0%**
Sodium 210mg	**9%**
Total Carbohydrate 26g	**9%**
Dietary Fiber 1g	**3%**
Sugars 11g	
Protein 2g	

Vitamin A 0%	•	Vitamin C 0%
Calcium 2%	•	Iron 8%

* Percent Daily Values are based on a 2,000 calorie diet. Your daily values may be higher or lower depending on your calorie needs:

	Calories:	2,000	2,500
Total Fat	Less than	65g	80g
Sat Fat	Less than	20g	25g
Cholesterol	Less than	300mg	300mg
Sodium	Less than	2400mg	2400mg
Total Carbohydrate		300g	375g
Dietary Fiber		25g	30g

Calories per gram:
Fat 9 • Carbohydrate 4 • Protein 4

After checking to see that the product contains under 450 milligrams of sodium per serving, check the amount of fat grams in the product. If it's less than 30 percent, according to the ratio of total amount of calories from fat, you can buy it.

Note the fat content on the graham cracker label above. Five crackers will give you 3 grams of fat. When 30 grams is your daily allowance, it's your personal decision as to whether these five crackers are worth it. Take a look at the sugars count: 11 grams. Is this less than one-third of the total carbohydrates? 26 carbohydrate grams ÷ 3 = 8.66 grams. 11 grams of sugars is over the limit, therefore this product is too high in sugars.

Use this knowledge to your advantage. Don't let foods with a high sodium, sugar, or fat content into your house! By doing this you will have won half the battle.

THE 1-2-3 NEVER SAY DIET QUICK LABEL TEST

1. Over 450 mg of sodium per serving? If so—DON'T BUY IT!
2. Simple sugars over 1/3 of total carbohydrates? If so— DON'T BUY IT!
3. Grams of fat per serving—is it worth it out of your daily 30-gram fat allowance? If not—DON'T BUY IT!

Also, with regard to nutritional facts and how to read the new food labels, check Appendix III at the end of the book. It provides even more detail to help you with the new nutritional labeling which went into effect on December 31, 1993.

Chapter Nine:

HOLIDAYS AND SPECIAL EVENTS: CELEBRATING IN HEALTHY STYLE

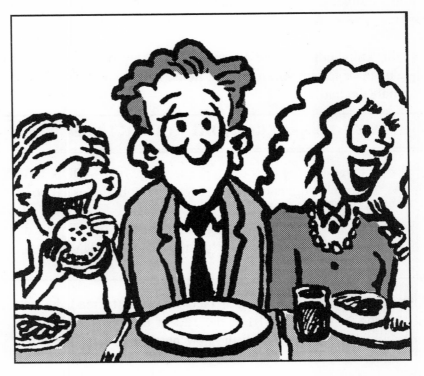

One of the main problems in trying to regulate weight control is maintaining healthy eating habits when attending special events. Major feasts are a traditional part of celebrating Thanksgiving, Easter, Christmas, the Fourth of July, Rosh Hashanah, Passover, weddings, anniversaries, and birthdays, etc. Unfortunately, many of us attend at least twenty to thirty of these events per year.

We also dine in restaurants with friends on occasions that are not major events at all—merely excuses to indulge in good food and pleasant conversation. We have to learn how to deal with these situations, otherwise whatever we do to regulate weight control won't be nearly enough.

As an example of how we can integrate everything we've learned in the Anti-Diet program to a special event, let's go to the typical Thanksgiving family dinner.

Our guidelines for proper eating habits as stated ealier, include eating four to six times a day. That program doesn't vary until we get to the actual Thanksgiving dinner itself. For example, if this meal is to begin at 3:00 p.m., maintain your regular schedule, starting with a normal breakfast between 6:00 and 9:00 a.m. Eat a piece of fruit for a snack before lunch, and, believe it or not, at 12:30 or 1:00 p.m. I will sit down and eat lunch. I will eat a bowl of rice with vegetables, or perhaps just a bowl of salad with soup, or any one of your regular lunches.

At this point you will have eaten three times. Your satiety center has received an indication that there is sugar in the body, and will slowly suppress hunger throughout the morning hours all the way till 2:00 P.M. When you sit down with the family for Thanksgiving dinner at 3:00, you will literally not be hungry.

Although you are not hungry, the first thing to do is pick up a bowl of salad and a slice of bread. Now, after your breakfast, the morning snack, lunch, the post-lunch snack, as well as the salad and bread, you are definitely not hungry. Wait for fifteen to twenty minutes before eating again. While everyone is already working on their dinner plates, and, of course, nagging you as to why you're not eating, explain that you will eat soon, that you are just taking a break. When the waiting period (fifteen to twenty minutes) is over, fill up your dinner plate with small amounts of everything on the table, regardless whether or not it's a little higher in fat than usual.

There is turkey, sweet potato, mashed potato, a little gravy, vegetables, etc. Of course, since you're not hungry, you will have a hard time finishing that plate. If you do finish, that's OK too. But remember one thing from our guidelines: never, ever have a second helping.

Two hours later the table is clean, an array of cakes and pies are rolling in right in front of you. What do you do now? First, look carefully to see if there is any fruit on the table. If there is, please take a piece of fruit, or whatever there is from the fruit department, and enjoy it. Then take another fifteen- to twenty-minute break. After that waiting period you can go for your dessert.

So, instead of following your usual pattern (i.e., taking a bite of this and a bite of that, a sliver of one cake then a sliver of another cake), try something very simple. Look at all of the desserts—make sure you see all of them—and select the ONE that you love the most. It doesn't matter how much fat is in it. It doesn't matter how much sugar is in it. Just pick out that special one. Cut yourself a normal slice, like any other guest at the table. Please eat it and enjoy it, without any feelings of guilt.

So what happened to you at this event? You might have eaten a little bit more this day, but you really did not indulge. You had breakfast, a piece of fruit, a small lunch, salad and bread, later on you had the dinner plate (after the waiting period), you ate a little more fruit, then after another waiting period you enjoyed dessert with a cup of coffee or tea or whatever. The end result was that you ate just a little too much today—not a lot, and probably over 30 grams of fat. However, with some advanced planning, a meal such as this can become part of your 300-Fat Pie system.

By regularly watching your fat intake through the Anti-Diet 300-Fat Pie system, you won't have a problem with holidays and events. Following the steps described in the Thanksgiving dinner, you will be able to celebrate with everyone else while maintaining your weight, regulating it in a better way, and sometimes even losing weight. I also recommend that you exercise on the day of an event— which means that you exercise in the morning. If you exercise three to five times per week, make sure you count the event day as one of those exercise days.

A different approach is to eat like anyone else around the table, knowing that this is the only day out of the plan that can rock your 300-fat pie. A friend who stopped by for family dinner introduced me to interesting concept: He had noticed that saying no to my mom for a second helping could start World War III, so his solution was to have a small first serving and a second one later—for world peace. One final alternative, for the athletic among us, just to keep the peaceful status-quo, is to eat double and exercise triple.

THE 10-STEP PLAN FOR HEALTHY HOLIDAY EATING

1. Exercise in the morning
2. Eat breakfast
3. Eat a pre-lunch snack (see list in Chapter Four)
4. Eat a regular lunch
5. At the special dinner, begin with a salad and piece of bread
6. Take a break for 15 to 20 minutes
7. Fill up your dinner plate ONCE with small amounts of whatever you like
8. Choose fruit for first dessert, if possible.
9. Take a break for 15 to 20 minutes
10. Enjoy ONE piece of whatever dessert you like

Some people utilizing this process of holiday and special event eating are able to lose weight during the ten-day period that includes the event. However, if you do not succeed in losing weight but maintain the same weight in that ten-day period, you are still doing very well. Following the event, you have the rest of the ten days to continue with the core of tthe Anti-Diet Plan.

NEVER DIET AGAIN!

I wish you a healthy life and good luck as you begin the exciting new changes that will affect your entire lifestyle. If you utilize the information provided in this book, you will never fall into the trap of traditional diets again. It is a privilege to share this vital information with you, and I thank you for buying this book, reading it, and, it is hoped, trying to implement it. In my experience with clients from all walks of life, the benefits of the Anti-Diet program will enhance total well-being. The benefits are many.

ANTI-DIET PROGRAM BENEFITS

<u>Nutritional</u> <u>Benefits</u>

- Offers an up-to-date education in good nutrition
- Propels correct eating habits and behavior
- Increases metabolism through eating and not dieting
- Provides a well-nourished food intake
- Because it's not a diet, the program:
    - eliminates deprivation
    - eliminates starvation
    - eliminates the need for measuring food
    - eliminates calorie counting

Activity Benefits

- Body fat loss
- Weight loss
- Increases muscular toning and strength
- Increases aerobic conditioning
- Increases bone density
- Increases metabolism
- Increases energy level
- Reduces stress
- Decreases probability for:
    - Heart disease
    - Stroke
    - Cancer
    - Diabetes
    - Hypertension
    - Hyperlipidemia
    - Slow down the osteoperosis process

Psychological Benefits

- Strengthens immune system
- Increases self-esteem
- Increases inner strength and motivation
- Reduces stress and depression
- Increases drive and perseverance
- Increases confidence

<u>Family</u> <u>Benefits</u>

- Maintains peace at home
- Keeps Mom smiling

I also invite you to feel free to contact me in writing with any questions you have about The Anti-Diet:

Dr. Mickey Harpaz
107 Newtown Road
Danbury, CT 06810

Appendix I:

SOURCES

Research studies regarding eating habits, proper nutrition, and active lifestyles that underly the Anti-Diet program have been published in The American Journal of Cardiology, The Journal of the American Medical Association, The Journal of the American Dietetic Association, Circulation (from The American Heart Association), and The Journal of the American College of Sports Medicine.

Dr. Mickey Harpaz regularly attends meetings and conferences of the American Heart Association, the American College of Sports Medicine, the American College of Cardiology, and the American Dietetic Association.

Appendix II:

ANTI-DIET CLIENT STORIES AND LETTERS

Mardi, who has lost 90 pounds on the Anti-Diet program, shares a story about his former lifestyle:

> Dear Dr. Harpaz:
>
> *I remember one time I went out to dinner with a vendor whom I dealt with. We went to this classy restaurant. This restaurant had chrome chairs. I felt mine weakening all night. I was afraid to lean back. Well, after the meal I felt like sitting back in the chair and guess what? The chair slowly collapsed, and I found myself on the floor unable to get up. The maitre d' tried to help me up with another waiter and everybody was watching. I was so embarrassed. After that I picked out my restaurants not by the food, but by the seats that they had. If they had the arm chair type of seats, I'd never go back—I just didn't fit. In fact, I even filled out a suggestion form at a certain hotel in Chicago to explain to them that it was almost discriminatory to have one*

*type of chair in the entire restaurant.
It discriminated against big people
like me who could not fit into any of
them. Guys, don't take for granted that
you are healthy. To you overweight
people, between us, get into proper
nutrition and an active lifestyle and
you can change the decision of which
restaurant you'd like to go to by the
menu, not the style of the chairs.*

One day Mardi decided to try my program. He educated himself about proper nutrition, how to eat healthfully, and how to begin exercising. Since then, Mardi has lost over 90 pounds and continues to lose weight. Many things are changing in his life, including tying his own shoelaces and being able, for the first time in his life, to sit on a plane in a window seat and eating normally on a tray that doesn't rest on his belly. He is now able to come to my office and sit on the sofa without having to think twice about being able to get up.

A recent letter sums up Mardi's experience since deciding to never diet again:

> ## Dear Mickey,
>
> *This is just a note to let you know how much I really appreciate all of the help you have given me in the past few months. I really had no understanding about why I was overweight or what I was eating, good or bad, or how it affected me mentally and physically. I have been to many doctors, dieticians and hospitals, all with very little success. If there was any success at all, it was very short-lived and I was quite miserable during the so-called "program."*
>
> *Mickey, you have given me my life back. Without your help in both nutrition and exercise programs I was headed for certain disaster. I never diet and still lose weight on your program. Moreover, I ate, six times a day, the foods that I enjoy, not the so-called "packaged foods" for health you hear so much about nowadays. You have given me an active lifestyle filled with education about nutrition and exercise that will be with me for the rest of my life.*
>
> *I thank you and my family thanks you.*

Tyrone, after successfully integrating the Anti-Diet program into his life, wrote me the following letter:

> Dear Mickey:
>
> *I would like to take this opportunity to extend my appreciation for the courtesy and excellent supervision provided to and for me during my use of your program. It is clear that unless such valuable direction is available, reaching desired goals relating to health, weight and nutrition will be much more difficult, if at all possible.*
>
> *My physician recommended a health club atmosphere to address general conditioning, weight and mental attitude. While ------ was my choice, I made little or no progress toward my goal, except superficial ones.*
>
> *Then I joined your program and within eight weeks had not only made a major impact in weight and general conditioning, but acquired direct health benefits in respect to a lung condition and an operation-affected muscle area. Perhaps the most significant benefit, if it were possible to single out one, would be the educational*

function. By learning about food and it's roles in my life from a nutritional and physiological standpoint, I was able to realign old eating habits. More importantly, I could make this adjustment with a positive attitude. The short-term benefits that come from this program are very rewarding and fulfill health needs in people's daily life—both physical and physiological.

In the final analysis, though it is due to the long-term benefits of sustained nutrition, good eating habits and a balanced attitude towards exercise will prove to be the real gift. All of this is only possible because of your program's deep commitment to integrate awareness through education in your clients. I would recommend this program to all who would want to improve their understanding of how to live better and healthier.

Joseph made healthy lifestyle changes with the Anti-Diet program to counteract his weight problem and a serious pulmonary condition. His letter is addressed to the director of the health club where I conducted my program:

I now have a new lease on life. I'm sure that you would like to know that this is due to Mickey Harpaz and his program, which is offered through your services. I'm sixty years old and for the past ten years I've been suffering with a chronic condition diagnosed as COPD [Chronic Obstructive Pulmonary Disease]. This, combined with my overweight and sporadic exercise program left me out of breath most of the time.

My daughter, who is an exercise physiologist in Florida, recommended that I look for a pulmonary program in my area. I was fortunate to find such a program being offered through your club. I would like you to know that Mickey Harpaz is an intelligent and sensitive person who offers an outstanding program. After six weeks I've lost eighteen pounds and am feeling much more physically fit and breathing better than I have in many years.

At this point in time I feel that Mickey has set some realistic goals for me and is giving me the knowledge and encouragement to move towards my goals.

Appendix III

THE U.S. LABELING LAW

The New Food Label at a Glance

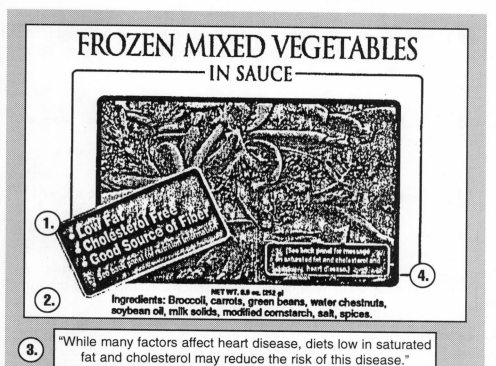

"While many factors affect heart disease, diets low in saturated fat and cholesterol may reduce the risk of this disease."

① **Descriptors:** While descriptive terms like "low," "good source," and "free" have long been used on food labels, their meaning – and their usefulness in helping consumers plan a healthy diet – have been murky. Now FDA has set specific definitions for these terms, assuring shoppers that they can believe what they read on the package:

- free
- light
- more
- good source

- high
- low
- reduced
- less

For fish, meat and poultry:

- lean
- extra lean

2. **Ingredients** still will be listed in descending order by weight, and now the list will be required on almost all foods, even standardized ones like mayonnaise and bread.

3. **Health claim message** referred to on the front panel is shown here.

4. **Health Claims:** For the first time, food labels will be allowed to carry the information about the link between certain nutrients and specific diseases. For such a "health claim" to be made on a package, the Food and Drug Administration must first determine that the diet-disease link is supported by scientific evidence. At this time, FDA is allowing seven specific claims about the relationships between:

- fat and cancer risk;
- saturated fat and cholesterol and heart disease risk;
- calcium and osteoporosis risk;
- sodium and hypertension risk;
- fruits, vegetables and grains that contain soluble fiber and heart disease risk;
- fiber-containing grain products, fruits and vegetables and cancer risk;
- fruits and vegetables and cancer risk.

Author's note: The following has been excerpted from the FDA's *Backgrounder* newsletter describing "The New Food Label." I apologize for the imperfect reproduction quality, but I feel the information that follows is important enough to be reprinted poorly rather than not at all.

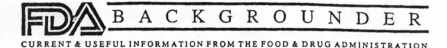

FDA BACKGROUNDER

CURRENT & USEFUL INFORMATION FROM THE FOOD & DRUG ADMINISTRATION

Grocery store aisles are on their way to becoming avenues to greater nutritional knowledge.

The new food label will make it possible. Under new regulations from the Food and Drug Administration of the Department of Health and Human Services and the Food Safety and Inspection Service of the U.S. Department of Agriculture, the food label will soon offer more complete, useful and accurate nutrition information than ever before.

The purpose of food label reform is simple: to clear up confusion that has prevailed on supermarket shelves for years, to help consumers choose more healthful diets, and to offer an incentive to food companies to improve the nutritional qualities of their products.

Among key changes taking place are:

• nutrition labeling for almost all foods. Consumers now will be able to learn about the nutritional qualities of almost all of the products they buy.

• information on the amount per serving of saturated fat, cholesterol, dietary fiber, and other nutrients that are of major health concern to today's consumers

• nutrient reference values, expressed as Percent of Daily Values, that can help consumers see how a food fits into an overall daily diet

• uniform definitions for terms that describe a food's nutrient content—such as "light," "low-fat," and "high-fiber"—to ensure that such terms mean the same for any product on

91

which they appear. These descriptors will be particularly helpful for consumers trying to moderate their intake of calories or fat and other nutrients, or for those trying to increase their intake of certain nutrients, such as fiber.

• claims about the relationship between a nutrient and a disease, such as calcium and osteoporosis, and fat and cancer. These will be helpful for people who are concerned about eating foods that may help keep them healthier longer.

• standardized serving sizes that make nutritional comparisons of similar products easier

• declaration of total percentage of juice in juice drinks. This will enable consumers to know exactly how much juice is in a product.

• voluntary nutrition information for many raw foods.

NLEA

These and other changes are part of final rules to be published soon in the *Federal Register*. FDA's rules meet the provisions of the Nutrition Labeling and Education Act of 1990 (NLEA), which, among other things, requires nutrition labeling for most foods (except meat and poultry) and authorizes the use of nutrient content claims and appropriate FDA-approved health claims.

Meat and poultry products regulated by USDA are not

covered by NLEA. However, USDA's regulations closely parallel FDA's new rules, summarized here.

Effective Dates

The new label may start to appear on products soon, although manufacturers have until May 1994 to comply with most of the new labeling requirements. Regulations pertaining to health claims and some parts of the ingredient labeling rule become effective in May 1993.

As provided by Congress under NLEA, FDA extended the implementation date for mandatory nutrition labeling and nutrient content descriptors by one year from the law's target date of May 1993 because of "undue economic hardship" that the earlier effective date would have caused.

Nutrition Labeling—Applicable Foods

The new regulations will require nutrition labeling on most foods. In addition, nutrition information currently is voluntary for many raw foods: the 20 most frequently eaten fresh fruits and vegetables and raw fish, under FDA's voluntary point-of-purchase nutrition information program. In fact, point-of-purchase information for raw produce and raw fish has been available in some grocery stores since November 1991.

Although voluntary, the programs for raw produce and raw meat, fish and poultry carry strong incentives for retailers to participate. The NLEA states that if voluntary compliance is insufficient, nutrition information for such raw foods will become mandatory.

Nutrition Labeling—Exemptions

Under NLEA, some foods are exempt from nutrition labeling. These include:
- food produced by small businesses (that is, those with food sales of less than $50,000 a year or total sales of less than $500,000)
- restaurant food
- food served for immediate consumption, such as that served in hospital cafeterias and airplanes
- ready-to-eat food prepared primarily on site; for example, bakery, deli, and candy store items
- food sold by food service vendors, such as mall cookie counters, sidewalk vendors, and vending machines
- food shipped in bulk, as long as it is not for sale in that form to consumers
- medical foods, such as those used to address the nutritional needs of patients with certain diseases
- plain coffee and tea, some spices, and other foods that contain no significant amounts of any nutrients

Although these foods are exempt, they are free to carry nutrition information, when appropriate—as long as it complies with the new regulations.

Also, packages with less than 12 square inches available for labeling do not have to carry nutrition information. However, they must provide an address or telephone number for consumers to obtain the required nutrition information.

Nutrition information about game meats—such as deer, bison, rabbit, quail, wild turkey, and ostrich—may be provided on counter cards, signs, or other point-of-purchase materials rather than on individual labels. Because little nutrient data exists for these foods, FDA believes that allowing this option will enable game meat producers to give first priority to collecting appropriate data and make it easier for them to update the information as it becomes available.

Nutrition Panel—Content

The new food label will feature a revamped nutrition panel. It will be headed with a new title, "Nutrition Facts," which replaces "Nutrition Information Per Serving." The new name will signal to consumers that the product label meets the new regulations.

There will be a new set of dietary components on the nutrition panel. The mandatory (underlined) and voluntary components and the order in which they must appear are:

- total calories
- calories from fat
- calories from saturated fat
- total fat
- saturated fat
- polyunsaturated fat
- monounsaturated fat
- cholesterol
- sodium
- potassium
- total carbohydrate
- dietary fiber
- soluble fiber
- insoluble fiber

- sugars
- sugar alcohol (for example, the sugar substitutes xylitol, mannitol and sorbitol)
- other carbohydrate (the difference between total carbohydrate and the sum of dietary fiber, sugars, and sugar alcohol if declared)
- protein
- vitamin A
- vitamin C
- calcium
- iron
- other essential vitamins and minerals

If a claim is made about any of the optional components, or if a food is fortified or enriched with any of them, nutrition information for these components then becomes mandatory.

These mandatory and voluntary components are the only ones allowed on the nutrition panel. The listing of single amino acids, maltodextrin, calories from polyunsaturated fat, and calories from carbohydrates, for example, may not appear as part of the nutrition facts on the label.

The required nutrients were selected because they address today's health concerns. The order in which they must appear reflects the priority of current dietary recommendations.

Thiamin, riboflavin and niacin will no longer be required in nutrition labeling because deficiencies of each are no longer considered of public health significance. However, they may be listed voluntarily.

Nutrition Panel—Format

The format for declaring nutrient content per serving also has been revised. Now, all nutrients must be declared as a percent of their Daily Value—the new label reference values. The amount, in grams, of macronutrients (such as fat, cholesterol, sodium, carbohydrates and protein) still must be listed to the immediate right of each of the names of each of these nutrients. But, for the first time, a column headed "% Daily Value" will appear, as will a footnote to help consumers place their individual nutrient needs with respect to the Daily Values used on the label.

Requiring nutrients to be declared as a percent of the Daily Value is intended to prevent misinterpretations that arise with quantitative values. For example, a food with 140 milligrams (mg) of sodium could be mistaken for a high-sodium food because 140 is a relatively large number. In actuality, however, that amount represents less than 6 percent of the Daily Value for sodium, which is 2,400 mg.

On the other hand, a food with 5 grams (g) of saturated fat could be construed as being low in that nutrient. But, in fact, that food would provide one-fourth the total Daily Value because 20 g is the Daily Value for saturated fat based on a 2,000-calorie diet.

Format Modifications

Variations in the format of the nutrition panel are allowed. Some are mandatory. For example, the labels of foods for children under 2 (except infant formula, which has special labeling rules under the Infant Formula Act of 1980) may not carry information about saturated fat, polyunsaturated fat, monounsaturated fat, cholesterol, calories from fat, or calories from saturated fat.

The reason is to prevent parents from wrongly assuming that infants and toddlers should restrict their fat intake, when, in fact, they should not. Fat is important during these years to ensure adequate growth and development.

Also, the labels of foods for children under 4 may not include the percent of Daily Values per serving or the actual Daily Values for macronutrients. Only the percent of the Daily Values for vitamins and minerals is allowed. The reason: FDA has not established Daily Values for macronutrients for this age group.

Some foods may qualify for a simplified label format. This format is allowed when the food contains insignificant amounts of seven or more of the mandatory nutrients and total calories. "Insignificant" means that a declaration of zero could be made in nutrition labeling, or, for total carbohydrate, dietary fiber, and protein, the declaration states "less than 1 g."

For foods for children under 2, the simplified format may be used if the product contains insignificant amounts of six or more of the following: calories, total fat, sodium, total carbohydrate, dietary fiber, sugars, protein, vitamins A and C, calcium, and iron.

If the simplified format is used, information on total calories, total fat, total carbohydrate, protein, and sodium—even if they are present in insignificant amounts—must be listed. Other nutrients, along with calories from fat, must be shown if they are present in more than insignificant amounts. Nutrients added to the food must be listed, too.

Small and medium-size packages will be granted certain exceptions to make the nutrition labeling practical on the smaller space.

Serving Sizes

Whatever the format, the serving size remains the basis for reporting each food's nutrient content. However, unlike in the past, when the serving size was up to the discretion of the food manufacturer, serving sizes now will be more uniform and will reflect the amounts that people actually eat. They also must be expressed in both common household and metric measures.

NLEA defines serving size as the amount of food customarily eaten at one time. The serving sizes that appear on food labels will be based on FDA-established lists of "Reference Amounts Customarily Consumed Per Eating Occasion."

These reference amounts, which are part of the new regulations, are broken down into 139 FDA-regulated food product categories, including 11 groups of foods specially formulated or processed for infants or children under 4. They list the amounts of food customarily consumed per eating occasion for each category, based primarily on national food consumption surveys. FDA's list also gives the suggested label statement for serving size declaration. For example, the category "breads (excluding sweet quick type), rolls" has a reference amount of 50 grams, and the appropriate label statement for sliced bread or roll is "__ piece(s) (__ g)" or, for unsliced bread, "2 oz (56 g/_ inch slice)."

The serving size of products that come in discrete units, such as cookies, candy bars and sliced products, is the number of whole units that most closely approximates the reference amount. Cookies are an example. Under the "bakery products" category, cookies have a reference amount of 30 g. The household measure closest to that amount is the number of cookies that comes closest to weighing 30 g. Thus, the serving size on the label of a package of cookies in which each cookie weighs 13 g would read "2 cookies (26 g)."

If one unit weighs more than 50 percent but less than 200 percent of the reference amount, the serving size is one unit. For example, the reference amount for bread is 50 g; therefore, the label of a loaf of bread in which each slice weighs more than 25 g would state a serving size of one slice.

Certain rules apply to food products that are packaged and sold individually. If such an individual package is less than 200 percent of the applicable reference amount, the item qualifies as one serving. Thus, a 360-milliliter (12-fluid-ounce) can of soda is one serving, since the reference amount for carbonated beverages is 240 mL (8 ounces).

However, if the product has a reference amount of 100 g or 100 mL or more and the package contains more than 150 percent but less than 200 percent of the reference amount, manufacturers have the option of deciding whether the product can be one or two servings.

An example is a 15-ounce (420 g) can of soup. The serving size reference amount for soup is 245 g. Therefore, the manufacturer has the option to declare the can of soup as one or two servings.

Daily Value—DRVs

The new label reference value, Daily Value (DV), comprises two new sets of dietary standards: Daily Reference Values (DRVs) and Reference Daily Intakes (RDIs). Only the Daily Value term will appear on the label, though, to make label reading less confusing.

As part of new regulations, DRVs are being introduced for macronutrients that are sources of energy: fat, carbohydrate (including fiber), and protein; and for cholesterol, sodium and potassium, which do not contribute calories.

DRVs for the energy-producing nutrients are based on the number of calories consumed per day. A daily intake of 2,000 calories has been established as the reference. This level was chosen because it has the greatest public health benefit for the nation.

DRVs for the energy-producing nutrients are calculated as follows:

• fat based on 30 percent of calories
• saturated fat based on 10 percent of calories
• carbohydrate based on 60 percent of calories
• protein based on 10 percent of calories. (The DRV for protein applies only to adults and children over 4. RDIs for protein for special groups have been established.)
• fiber based on 11.5 g of fiber per 1,000 calories.

Because of current public health recommendations, DRVs for some nutrients represent the uppermost limit that is considered desirable. The DRVs for fats and sodium are:

• total fat: less than 65 g
• saturated fat: less than 20 g
• cholesterol: less than 300 mg
• sodium: less than 2,400 mg

Daily Value—RDIs

The RDI replaces the term "U.S. RDA," which was introduced in 1973 as a label reference value for vitamins, minerals and protein in voluntary nutrition labeling. The name change was sought because of confusion that existed over "U.S. RDAs," the values determined by FDA and used on food labels, and "RDAs" (Recommended Dietary Allowances), the values determined by the National Academy of Sciences for various population groups and used by FDA to figure the U.S. RDAs.

However, the values for the new RDIs will remain the same as the old U.S. RDAs for the time being. Under the provisions of the Dietary Supplement Act of 1992, FDA plans to propose after Dec. 31, 1993, new values for the RDIs.

Nutrient Content Descriptors

The new regulations also spell out what terms may be used to describe the level of a nutrient in a food and how they can be used. These are the core terms:

• *Free.* This term means that a product contains no amount of, or only trivial or "physiologically inconsequential" amounts of, one or more of these components: fat, saturated fat, cholesterol, sodium, sugars, and calories. For example, "calorie-free" means fewer than 5 calories per serving and "sugar-free" and "fat-free" both mean less than 0.5 g per serving. Synonyms for "free" include "without," "no" and "zero."

• *Low.* This term could be used on foods that could be eaten frequently without exceeding dietary guidelines for one or more of these components: fat, saturated fat, cholesterol, sodium, and calories. Thus, descriptors would be defined as follows:

  • *low fat:* 3 g or less per serving
  • *low saturated fat:* 1 g or less per serving
  • *low sodium:* less than 140 mg per serving
  • *very low sodium:* less than 35 mg per serving
  • *low cholesterol:* less than 20 mg per serving
  • *low calorie:* 40 calories or less per serving.

Synonyms for low include "little," "few," and "low source of."

• *Lean and extra lean.* These terms can be used to describe the fat content of meat, poultry, seafood, and game meats.

  • *lean:* less than 10 g fat, less than 4 g saturated fat, and less than 95 mg cholesterol per serving and per 100 g.
  • *extra lean:* less than 5 g fat, less than 2 g saturated fat, and less than 95 mg cholesterol per serving and per 100 g.

• *High.* This term can be used if the food contains 20 percent or more of the Daily Value for a particular nutrient in a serving.

• *Good source.* This term means that one serving of a food contains 10 to 19 percent of the Daily Value for a particular nutrient.

• *Reduced.* This term means that a nutritionally altered product contains 25 percent less of a nutrient or of calories than the regular, or reference, product. However, a reduced claim can't be made on a product if its reference food already meets the requirement for a "low" claim.

• *Less.* This term means that a food, whether altered or not, contains 25 percent less of a nutrient or of calories than the reference food. For example, pretzels that have 25 percent less fat than potato chips could carry a "less" claim. "Fewer" is an acceptable synonym.

• *Light.* This descriptor can mean two things:

First, that a nutritionally altered product contains one-third fewer calories or half the fat of the reference food. If the food derives 50 percent or more of its calories from fat, the reduction must be 50 percent of the fat.

Second, that the sodium content of a low-calorie, low-fat food has been reduced by 50 percent. In addition, "light in sodium" may be used on food in which the sodium content has been reduced by at least 50 percent.

The term "light" still can be used to describe such properties as texture and color, as long as the label explains the intent; for example, "light brown sugar" and "light and fluffy."

• *More.* This term means that a serving of food, whether altered or not, contains a nutrient that is at least 10 percent of the Daily Value more than the reference food. The 10 percent of Daily Value also would apply to "fortified," "enriched" and "added" claims, but in those cases, the food must be altered.

Other Definitions

The regulations also address other claims. Among them:

• *Percent fat free:* A product bearing this claim must be a low-fat or a fat-free product. In addition, the claim must accurately reflect the amount of fat present in 100 g of the food. Thus, if a food contains 2.5 g fat per 50 g, the claim must be "95 percent fat free."

• *Implied:* These types of claims are prohibited when they wrongfully imply that a food contains or does not contain a meaningful level of a nutrient. For example, a product claiming to be made with an ingredient known to be a source of fiber (such as "made with oat bran") is not allowed unless the product contains enough of that ingredient (for example, oat bran) to meet the definition for "good source" of fiber. As another example, a claim that a product contains "no tropical oils" is allowed—but only on foods that are "low" in saturated fat because consumers have come to equate tropical oils with high saturated fat.

• *Meals and main dishes:* Claims that a meal or main dish is "free" of a nutrient, such as sodium or cholesterol, must meet the same requirements as those for individual foods. Other claims can be used under special circumstances. For example, "low-calorie" means the meal or main dish contains 120 calories or less per 100 g. "Low-sodium" means the food has 140 mg or less per 100 g. "Low-cholesterol" means the food contains 20 mg cholesterol or less per 100 g and no more than 2 g saturated fat. "Light" means the meal or main dish is low-fat or low-calorie.

• *Standardized foods:* Any nutrient content claim, such as "reduced fat," "low calorie," and "light," may be used in conjunction with a standardized term if the new product has been specifically formulated to meet FDA's criteria for that claim, if the product is not nutritionally inferior to the traditional standardized food, and the new product complies with certain compositional requirements set by FDA. A new product bearing a claim also must have performance characteristics similar to the referenced traditional standardized food. If the product doesn't, and the differences materially limit the product's use, its label must state the differences (for example, not recommended for baking) to inform consumers.

• *Healthy:* FDA also is issuing a proposal to define the term "healthy." Under that proposal, "healthy" could be used to describe a food that is low in fat and saturated fat and contains no more than 480 mg sodium and no more than 60 mg cholesterol per serving. A final rule is expected in 1993.

"Fresh"

Although not mandated by NLEA, FDA also issued a regulation for the term "fresh." The agency took this step because of concern over the term's possible misuse on some food labels.

The regulation defines the term "fresh" when it is used to suggest that a food is raw or unprocessed. In this context, "fresh" can be used only on a food that is raw, has never been frozen or heated, and contains no preservatives. (Irradiation at low levels is allowed.) "Fresh frozen," "frozen fresh," and "freshly frozen" can be used for foods that are

Other uses of the term "fresh," such as in "fresh milk" or "freshly baked bread," are not affected.

Baby Foods

FDA is not allowing broad use of nutrient claims on infant and toddler foods. However, the agency may propose later claims specifically for these foods. The terms "unsweetened" and "unsalted" are allowed on these foods, however, because they relate to taste and not nutrient content.

Health Claims

Claims for seven relationships between a nutrient or a food and the risk of a disease or health-related condition will be allowed for the first time. They can be made in several ways: through third-party references, such as the National Cancer Institute; statements; symbols, such as a heart; and vignettes or descriptions. Whatever the case, the claim must meet the requirements for authorized health claims; for example, they cannot state the degree of risk reduction and can only use "may" or "might" in discussing the nutrient or food-disease relationship. And they must state that other factors play a role in that disease.

They also must be phrased so that the consumer can understand the relationship between the nutrient and the disease and the nutrient's importance in relationship to a daily diet.

An example of an appropriate claim is: "While many factors affect heart disease, diets low in saturated fat and cholesterol may reduce the risk of this disease."

The allowed nutrient-disease relationship claims and rules for their use are:

• *Calcium and osteoporosis:* To carry this claim, a food must contain 20 percent or more of the DV for calcium (200 mg) per serving, have a calcium content that equals or exceeds the food's content of phosphorus, and contain a form of calcium that can be readily absorbed and used by the body. The claim must name the target group most in need of adequate calcium intakes (that is, teens and young adult white and Asian women) and state the need for exercise and a healthy diet. A product that contains 40 percent or more of the DV for calcium must state on the label that a total dietary intake greater than 200 percent of the DV for calcium (that is, 2,000 mg or more) has no further known benefit.

• *Fat and cancer:* To carry this claim, a food must meet the descriptor requirements for "low-fat," or, if fish and game meats, for "extra lean."

• *Saturated fat and cholesterol and coronary heart disease (CHD):* This claim may be used if the food meets the definitions for the descriptors "low saturated fat," "low-cholesterol," and "low-fat," or, if fish and game meats, for "extra lean." It may mention the link between reduced risk of CHD and lower saturated fat and cholesterol intakes to lower blood cholesterol levels.

• *Fiber-containing grain products, fruits and vegetables and cancer:* To carry this claim, a food must be or must contain a grain product, fruit or vegetable and meet the descriptor requirements for "low-fat," and, without fortification, be a "good source" of dietary fiber.

• *Fruits, vegetables and grain products that contain fiber and risk of CHD:* To carry this claim, a food must be or must contain fruits, vegetables and grain products. It also must meet the descriptor requirements for "low saturated fat," "low-cholesterol," and "low-fat" and contain, without fortification, at least 0.6 g soluble fiber per serving.

• *Sodium and hypertension (high blood pressure):* To carry this claim, a food must meet the descriptor requirements for "low-sodium."

• *Fruits and vegetables and cancer:* This claim may be made for fruits and vegetables that meet the descriptor requirements for "low-fat" and that, without fortification, for "good source" of at least one of the following: dietary fiber or vitamins A or C. This claim relates diets low in fat and rich in fruits and vegetables (and thus vitamins A and C and dietary fiber) to reduced cancer risk. FDA authorized this claim in place of an antioxidant vitamin and cancer claim.

Folic Acid

In its soon-to-be published rules, FDA is denying the use of a health claim for folic acid and neural tube defects. In September 1992, the U.S. Public Health Service recommended that all women of childbearing age consume 0.4 mg of folic acid daily to reduce their risk of having a pregnancy affected with a neural tube defect. PHS identified several issues that remain to be resolved before FDA can take appropriate action to implement the recommendation and to decide whether to authorize a claim. The issues include the appropriate level of folic acid in food, safety concerns regarding increased intakes of folic acid, and specific options for implementation.

In November 1992, FDA convened an advisory committee to consider these issues. FDA is now reviewing that committee's recommendations.

Ingredient Labeling

As part of the new rules, the list of ingredients will undergo some changes, too. Chief among them is a new regulation that requires full ingredient labeling on "standardized foods," which previously were exempt. Ingredient declaration will now have to be on all foods that have more than one ingredient.

Also, the ingredient list will include, when appropriate:
• FDA-certified color additives, such as FD&C Blue No. 1, by name
• sources of protein hydrolysates, which are used in many foods as flavors and flavor enhancers
• declaration of caseinate as a milk derivative in the ingredient list of foods that claim to be non-dairy, such as coffee whiteners

The main reason for these new requirements is that some people may be allergic to such additives and will now be better able to avoid them.

As required by NLEA, beverages that claim to contain juice now must declare the total percentage of juice on the information panel. In addition, FDA's regulation establishes criteria for naming juice beverages. For example, when the label of a multi-juice beverage states one or more—but not all—of the juices present, and the predominantly named juice is present in minor amounts, the product's name must state that the beverage is flavored with that juice or declare the amount of the juice in a 5-percent range; for example, "raspberry flavored juice blend" or "juice blend, 2 to 7 percent raspberry juice."

Economic Impact

It is estimated that the new food label will cost FDA-regulated food processors between $1.4 billion and $2.3 billion over the next 20 years. The benefits to public health—measured in monetary terms—are estimated to well exceed the costs. Potential benefits include decreased rates of coronary heart disease, cancer, osteoporosis, obesity, high blood pressure, and allergic reactions to food.

Public Education

To help consumers get the most from the new food label, FDA and USDA have embarked on a multi-year food labeling education campaign. The campaign involves participation from consumer, trade and health groups, as well as other government agencies. Its purpose is to increase consumers' knowledge and effective use of the new food label and assist them in making accurate and sound dietary choices in accordance with the Dietary Guidelines for Americans.

Along with the new food label, education materials are expected to start making their appearance in early 1993.

Ordering *Federal Register* Documents

Reprints of the *Federal Register* document containing the regulations will be available for $4.50 a set from the U.S. Government Printing Office (GPO). Orders can be made by writing to the Superintendent of Documents, Washington, DC 20401, or calling (202) 783-3238, or faxing to (202) 512-2250. The GPO order number is 069-001-00045-9. Rush service will be available. Check, money order, VISA, and MasterCard are accepted.

Copies also will be available for sale at the main GPO bookstore at 710 North Capitol St., N.W., Washington, DC 20402.

Upon publication, the regulations also will be available on computer diskettes. A package of four diskettes with supplemental printed material will cost $88.50. Orders can be placed after publication by writing to the Superintendent of Documents or by calling GPO at (202) 512-1530 or faxing to (202) 512-1262. A limited number of diskettes also will be available for sale at the main GPO bookstore in Washington, D.C. To check on availability, call (202) 512-0132. Refer to order number 069-001-00046-7.

The documents also will be available on the Federal Bulletin Board for downloading by those who hold a Superintendent of Documents deposit account. To find out when the documents have been placed on the computer bulletin board, call (202) 512-1387.

Food Label Formats

1. PACKAGE LABELS OF **LESS THAN 12 SQUARE INCHES** MUST MEET THE FOLLOWING NUTRITION LABEL REQUIREMENT:

No Nutrition Label. Must display telephone number or address for consumer to call or write for nutrition information.

2. PACKAGE LABELS BETWEEN **12 AND 40 SQUARE INCHES** MUST MEET THE FOLLOWING MINIMUM NUTRITION LABEL REQUIREMENT:

INGREDIENTS: WHITE TUNA, WATER, VEGETABLE BROTH, HYDROLYZED CASEIN, HYDROLYZED SOY PROTEIN, SALT, PYROPHOSPHATE. DISTRIBUTOR **BUMBLE BEE**	**Nutrition Facts** Serv. Size 2 oz. (56 g/about ¼ cup) Servings about 2.5 **Calories** 60 Fat Cal. 10 *Percent Daily Values (DV) are based on a 2,000 calorie diet.	Amount / serving	%DV*	Amount / serving	%DV*
		Total Fat 1g	**2%**	**Total Carb.** 0g	**0%**
		Sat. Fat 0g	**0%**	Fiber 0g	**0%**
		Cholest. 25mg	**8%**	Sugars 0g	
		Sodium 250mg	**10%**	**Protein** 13g	**26%**
		Vitamin A 0% • Vitamin C 0% • Calcium 0% • Iron 0%			
		Niacin 20% • Vitamin B-6 8% • Vitamin B-12 10% • Phosphorus 8%			

3. PACKAGE LABELS OF **40 OR MORE SQUARE INCHES** MUST MEET THE FOLLOWING MINIMUM NUTRITION LABEL REQUIREMENT:

18% OF CALORIES FROM FAT

Nutrition Facts

Serving Size 1 Bar (28g)
Servings Per Container 10

Amount Per Serving

Calories 110   Calories from Fat 20

% Daily Value*

Total Fat 2g	**3%**
Saturated Fat 0.5g	**3%**
Cholesterol 0mg	**0%**
Sodium 100mg	**4%**
Total Carbohydrate 22g	**7%**
Dietary Fiber 1g	**4%**
Sugars 10g	
Protein 2g	

Iron	2%

Not a significant source of Vitamin A, Vitamin C, Calcium.
* Percent Daily Values are based on a 2,000 calorie diet.
Your daily values may be higher or lower depending on
your calorie needs:

	Calories:	2,000	2,500
Total Fat	Less than	65g	80g
Sat Fat	Less than	20g	25g
Cholesterol	Less than	300mg	300mg
Sodium	Less than	2,400mg	2,400mg
Total Carbohydrate		300g	375g
Dietary Fiber		25g	30g

Calories per gram:
Fat 9 • Carbohydrate 4 • Protein 4

4. PACKAGE LABELS FOR FOODS **CONTAINING LIMITED NUTRI-
ENTS** MAY USE A **SIMPLIFIED** FORMAT, E.G., FOR A SOFT DRINK:

Nutrition Facts

Serving Size 8 fl oz (240 mL)
Servings Per Container 2.5

Amount Per Serving

Calories 110

% Daily Value*

Total Fat 0g	**0%**
Sodium 50mg	**2%**
Total Carbohydrate 31g	**10%**
Sugars 31g	
Protein 0g	

*Percent Daily Values are based
on a 2,000 calorie diet.

Dr. Mickey Harpaz grew up in Israel, attended college in Wingate Institute (1974-1977), and then joined the Israel Defense Forces. Dr. Harpaz was an instructor of the Wingate Institute Army Base in Israel (1977-1979), and an officer trainer of pilots and officers in the Israeli Air Force (1979-1981).

Dr. Harpaz attended Adelphi University, N.Y., B.S. (1983), M.S. in Applied Physiology (1984), and Doctorate degree in Applied Physiology at Columbia University (1986-1993).

Dr. Harpaz gained hands-on experience at St. Mary's Hospital in New York city: In-Patients Quest for Disease Avoidance and Reconditioning (1985-1987).

Dr. Mickey Harpaz has been teaching and lecturing on physiology, weight control and health care issues. He has had his own radio talk show on health and fitness, and was the resident health consultant for Connecticut Independent Television Channel 20 WTXX talk show.

In his practice, Dr. Harpaz designs customized health programs that cover all issues that need to be addressed to maintain a healthy lifestyle. Depending on the specific requirements, the programs might be: cardiac recovery, cardiovascular health, weight control, proper nutrition and correct eating habits (1987-present)

Dr. Harpaz and his wife Jill were married in 1987. They have two sons, Aitan (b. 1991), and Koren (b. 1994). The Harpaz family lives in Brookfield, CT.